## Also Available From the American Academy of Pediatrics

ADHD: What Every Parent Needs to Know

Allergies and Asthma: What Every Parent Needs to Know

Autism Spectrum Disorder: What Every Parent Needs to Know

Baby and Toddler Basics: Expert Answers to Parents' Top 150 Questions

Baby Care Anywhere: A Quick Guide to Parenting On the Go

The Big Book of Symptoms: A–Z Guide to Your Child's Health

Building Resilience in Children and Teens: Giving Kids Roots and Wings

Caring for Your Baby and Young Child: Birth to Age 5*

Dad to Dad: Parenting Like a Pro

Food Fights: Winning the Nutritional Challenges of Parenthood Armed With Insight, Humor, and a Bottle of Ketchup

Guide to Toilet Training*

Heading Home With Your Newborn: From Birth to Reality

Mama Doc Medicine: Finding Calm and Confidence in Parenting, Child Health, and Work-Life Balance

My Child Is Sick! Expert Advice for Managing Common Illnesses and Injuries

New Mother's Guide to Breastfeeding*

Nutrition: What Every Parent Needs to Know

The Picky Eater Project: 6 Weeks to Happier, Healthier Family Mealtimes

Raising an Organized Child: 5 Steps to Boost Independence, Ease Frustration, and Promote Confidence

Raising Kids to Thrive: Balancing Love With Expectations and Protection With Trust

Retro Baby: Cut Back on All the Gear and Boost Your Baby's Development With More Than 100 Time-tested Activities

Retro Toddler: More Than 100 Old-School Activities to Boost Development

Sleep: What Every Parent Needs to Know

Understanding the NICU: What Parents of Preemies and Other Hospitalized Newborns Need to Know

Waking Up Dry: A Guide to Help Children Overcome Bedwetting

Your Baby's First Year*

**For additional parenting resources, visit the HealthyChildren bookstore at**
**http://shop.aap.org/for-parents.**

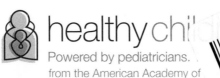 

healthy chi
Powered by pediatricians.
from the American Academy of

*This book is also available in Spanish.

Mom Pediatrician

# RAISING TWINS

### 3rd Edition

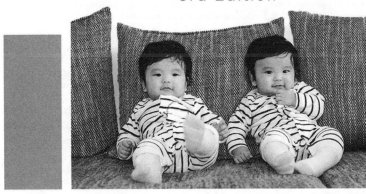

## Parenting Multiples
## From Pregnancy
## Through the School Years

Shelly Vaziri Flais, MD, FAAP

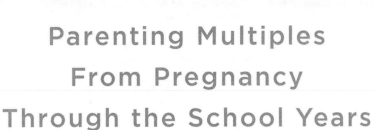

American Academy of Pediatrics
DEDICATED TO THE HEALTH OF ALL CHILDREN®

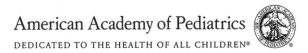

## American Academy of Pediatrics Publishing Staff

Mary Lou White, *Chief Product and Services Officer/SVP, Membership, Marketing, and Publishing*
Mark Grimes, *Vice President, Publishing*
Kathryn Sparks, *Manager, Consumer Publishing*
Shannan Martin, *Production Manager, Consumer Publications*
Amanda Helmholz, *Medical Copy Editor*
Peg Mulcahy, *Manager, Art Direction and Production*
Sara Hoerdeman, *Marketing Manager, Consumer Products*

Published by the American Academy of Pediatrics
345 Park Blvd
Itasca, IL 60143
Telephone: 630/626-6000
Facsimile: 847/434-8000
www.aap.org

The American Academy of Pediatrics is an organization of 67,000 primary care pediatricians, pediatric medical subspecialists, and pediatric surgical specialists dedicated to the health, safety, and well-being of infants, children, adolescents, and young adults.

The information contained in this publication should not be used as a substitute for the medical care and advice of your pediatrician. There may be variations in treatment that your pediatrician may recommend based on individual facts and circumstances.

Statements and opinions expressed are those of the author and not necessarily those of the American Academy of Pediatrics.

Any websites, brand names, products, or manufacturers are mentioned for informational and identification purposes only and do not imply an endorsement by the American Academy of Pediatrics (AAP). The AAP is not responsible for the content of external resources. Information was current at the time of publication.

The persons whose photographs are depicted in this publication are professional models. They have no relation to the issues discussed. Any characters they are portraying are fictional.

The publishers have made every effort to trace the copyright holders for borrowed materials. If they have inadvertently overlooked any, they will be pleased to make the necessary arrangements at the first opportunity.

This publication has been developed by the American Academy of Pediatrics. The contributors are expert authorities in the field of pediatrics. No commercial involvement of any kind has been solicited or accepted in development of the content of this publication. Disclosures: The author reports no disclosures.

Every effort is made to keep *Raising Twins* consistent with the most recent advice and information available from the American Academy of Pediatrics.

Special discounts are available for bulk purchases of this publication. Email Special Sales at aapsales@aap.org for more information.

Printed in the United States of America
9-424        1 2 3 4 5 6 7 8 9 10
CB0113
ISBN: 978-1-61002-333-7
eBook: 978-1-61002-334-4
EPUB: 978-1-61002-335-1
Kindle: 978-1-61002-336-8
PDF: 978-1-61002-337-5

Cover design by Daniel Rembert
Publication design by Linda Diamond
Illustrations by Tony LeTourneau

Library of Congress Control Number: 2018964823

# What People Are Saying About *Raising Twins*

—≈≈≈—

[Dr Flais'] empowering and confident tone is neighborly and down-to-earth, keeping parents attuned to her if-I-can-do-it-so-can-you attitude.
—*Publishers Weekly*

—≈≈≈—

Dr Flais has the experience and training as a mother of twins and a pediatrician to get it right. She knows how to double the joy of being a parent.
—Marc Weissbluth, MD, FAAP

Author of *Healthy Sleep Habits, Happy Child* and *Healthy Sleep Habits, Happy Twins*

—≈≈≈—

*Raising Twins: Parenting Multiples From Pregnancy Through the School Years,* 2nd Edition, by Shelly Vaziri Flais, MD, FAAP, is a book I wish I had when my multiples were younger. Raising multiples is a challenging task, and as the mother of 20-year-old fraternal girls and a teenage son, I have navigated more emotional waters than I want to remember! Through the support of my multiples club on the local and state levels, I found wise and helpful "anchors" to help me cope with those sometimes turbulent times. Dr Flais' book discusses how family dynamic changes when multiples arrive and offers insights on schedules, equipment, feedings, and other care issues. This must-have book contains indispensable information and guidance that mothers of multiples can reference for years. The perspective Dr Flais provides as a pediatrician and mother of twins is invaluable.
—Denise Anderson

Past president, Illinois Organization of Mothers of Twins Clubs, Inc

—≈≈≈—

Who better to hold your hand and help prepare you for the multiple joys (and challenges) of parenting twins than a pediatrician-mother of twins? By combining a medically sound foundation with a fully updated, reality-based approach, *Raising Twins* continues to provide new and expectant parents of twins a double dose of valuable advice and insight, while adding welcomed new and expanded second-edition insights including parenting premature infants and multiples.
—Laura A. Jana, MD, FAAP

Coauthor of *Heading Home With Your Newborn* and *Food Fights* and an identical twin!

—≈≈≈—

This book is chock-full of useful advice and comforting anecdotes for parents of multiples. I wish it had been on the bookshelf when I had mine!

—Gale Gand

Chef, author, and mother of twins

——∽∾∽——

Tandem feeding, duo sleeping, "twinproofing," and double discipline are only a few of the many tips on raising twins covered in this handy must-have parenting guide. Pediatrician and mom of twins, Dr Flais shares a double dose of practical information that I recommend all parents of multiples read before delivery and keep close at hand during the first few years.

—Tanya Altmann, MD, FAAP

Author of *Baby and Toddler Basics* and editor in chief of *Caring for Your Baby and Young Child*

——∽∾∽——

Double your pleasure but save time, stress, and money! *Raising Twins* helps parents of multiples hit the ground running and build their skills, efficiency, and confidence. A mom of twins and 2 singletons herself, Dr Flais also shares tips on celebrating your twins' "twinness"—as well as their individuality. This practical resource is a necessity for anyone caring for twins!

—Jennifer Shu, MD, FAAP

Coauthor of *Heading Home With Your Newborn* and *Food Fights*

——∽∾∽——

If you've just learned you're expecting twins or if you want strategies and tips from a mom of multiples who has been there, *Raising Twins* is the book you need. *Raising Twins* is an invaluable resource for any family with twins. Dr Flais gives detailed, practical strategies for gracefully handling the daily challenges of having multiple children of the same age (schedules, feeding, sleep training, discipline) and does it with the voice of experience. Knowing Dr Flais is not only a pediatrician but also a mother of 4 (including twins) made me sit up and listen to her practical tips. I especially appreciate her thoughts on the importance of nurturing and appreciating each child as an individual. The tone of the book is easy and conversational; you can tell Dr Flais is speaking from experience.

—Lisa Zollner

Attorney and mother of 3 (including twins)

——∽∾∽——

To all families with multiples and to my
beloved family.

Remember you are over the Edge of the Wild now,

and in for all sorts of fun wherever you go.

— Gandalf, *The Hobbit; or,*

*There and Back Again,*

by J.R.R. Tolkien

# Contents

# Please Note

The information and advice in this book apply equally to children and adolescents of both sexes except where noted. To indicate this, we have chosen to alternate between masculine pronouns and feminine pronouns throughout the book.

The American Academy of Pediatrics recognizes the diversity of lifestyles and family arrangements. Please note that this advice applies equally to parents, single-parent families, partners, spouses, grandparents, and others involved in caring for children and adolescents.

The information contained in this book is intended to complement, not be a substitute for, the advice of your pediatrician. Before starting any medical treatment or program, you should consult with your pediatrician, who can discuss your child's individual needs and advise you about symptoms and treatment. If you have any questions about how the information in this book applies to your child, speak with your pediatrician.

This book has been developed by the American Academy of Pediatrics. The contributors are expert authorities in the field of pediatrics. No commercial involvement of any kind has been solicited or accepted in the development of the content of this book.

# Acknowledgments

Years ago, when I began a journey to write a book about raising twins, I couldn't have imagined that one day I'd be putting together acknowledgments for the book's third edition. Any journey is done in baby steps, one day at a time, the same way parents navigate baby twins' first year.

I have many people to thank for playing a special role in the development of all of the editions of this book. The opportunity to write *Raising Twins* has been a complete joy and honor. It combines the passion I have as a pediatrician to help other parents raise their children happily and healthfully with the practical, real-world knowledge I have gained while raising twins in addition to single-born siblings close in age.

For all 3 editions, I thank Sarah Lacey Pilarowski, MD, FAAP, IBCLC, assistant clinical professor at the University of Colorado School of Medicine, Department of Pediatrics, and pediatrician at Sapphire Pediatrics for her invaluable peer review of book content, as well as a rewarding long-term friendship. I also thank Kristina Ferro Keating, MD, FAAP, partner at Lake Forest Pediatrics in Lake Forest, IL, for her invaluable peer review of book content and years of friendship.

Huge thanks to our wonderful team at the American Academy of Pediatrics (AAP) for their guidance and expertise—Mark Grimes, vice president of publishing, who has championed this book and mission since its conception on day 1; Kathryn Sparks, manager, consumer publishing; Jeff Mahony, director of professional and consumer publishing; and the entire production team. I also acknowledge Carolyn Kolbaba, former manager of AAP consumer publishing, for her particularly thorough and insightful involvement with the production of our first edition.

Over the years, my clinical pediatrics practice, Pediatric Health Associates, based in Naperville, IL, has cared for countless families with twins, triplets, and more. Thanks to the fact that I am a mom of twins and the author of the AAP book on raising twins, I care for quite a proportion of twins and triplets, which I find incredibly fulfilling. I thank my patients and their families not only for entrusting their care to me but also for continuing to teach me about parenting multiples. No two families are alike, and strategies need to be tweaked for the individual family's situation and that of each child. Thank you for being a daily reminder of this diversity within our community.

Matthew, Andrew, Ryan, and Nancy—you are each remarkable, unique individuals whose presence makes this world a better place. Years ago, I lovingly told my son Ryan, "There is no one like you," and he paused and responded ironically, "What about Andrew?" Such a funny moment, and it underscores that I take their individuality truly to heart. To Mike, raising twins and more is truly a team effort; we went from 2-on-1 to zone defense in a single pregnancy, so thank you for being a team player. As Captain Scott Kelly says, "Teamwork makes the dream work."

A hearty thanks to the numerous wonderful families with multiples who helpfully shared their thoughts, experiences, and notes with me during the process of writing all 3 editions of this book:

| | | |
|---|---|---|
| Adler Family | Graf Family | Long Family |
| Ali Family | Greenawalt Family | Morris Family |
| Anonymous families | Hartman Family | Orrico Family |
| Bell Family | Henderson Family | Peters Family |
| Buteau/Erickson Family | Hepokoski Family | Rappoport Family |
| Coleman Family | Hoff Family | Ramaswamy Family |
| Colley Family | Hynek Family | Sayles Family |
| DeGuzman Family | Irhke Family | Scheidler Family |
| Derk Family | Jablonski Family | Slinde Family |
| DeRome Family | Janson Family | Styzcen Family |
| Didrickson Family | Scott (and Mark) Kelly | Vervack Family |
| Dooyema Family | Kowynia Family | Winkler Family |
| DuMais Family | LaMonte Family | Zollner Family |
| Fraser Family | Lange Family | |

And I thank you, our readers. Congratulations on joining our ranks of families with multiples! Our multiples community is incredibly supportive of one another through all the challenges and triumphs of parenting twins, triplets, and more. You will learn much about parenting multiples; please pay it forward and share this knowledge with others. In *Star Wars: Episode VI—Return of the Jedi,* Yoda asked of Luke Skywalker, a well-known twin, "Pass on what you have learned." Spread the love and pass on the lessons you have learned to other families with multiples.

# CHAPTER 1

# A New Adventure

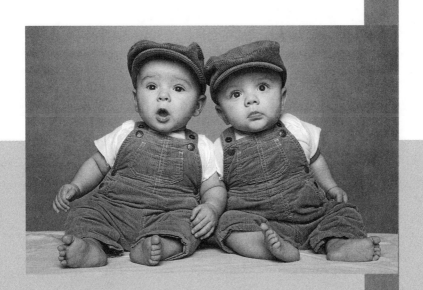

M om, can Andrew and I practice driving the car this weekend?" Ryan asked.

My identical twin sons, Andrew and Ryan, are growing up faster than I could have imagined. It seems only a few weeks ago that I saw 2 heartbeats on the ultrasound screen, learning I was pregnant with twins 16 years ago, and only yesterday that we removed the training wheels from their bicycles and watched them whiz by us, confident and elated with their new freedom.

Now, yet again, I'm feeling that roller-coaster sensation of watching our sons take yet another leap forward toward greater independence. Were they ready? Were *we* ready?

"Yes, Ryan, that's a great idea," I said, feeling a mix of emotions common to all parents—trepidation combined with love and pride. Our family has reached yet another milestone as our twins make their way forward on their unique paths into adulthood.

## Your New Life With Multiples

If you are expecting or are already parenting twins, triplets, or more, congratulations! If you are nervous about the challenges of raising multiples, remain calm and take a deep breath. With preparation, planning, organization, and the support of those around you, you can do this. Feeling unsure about parenting multiples is natural because it is a completely new experience and responsibility. That said, you will surprise yourself with your ability to adapt to your new family dynamic. The first year or so with twins is spent synchronizing your babies' schedules to make life easier. As your multiples grow, you will nurture each of them as an individual. In the blink of an eye, your children will ride their bikes in figure-eight patterns around you. In 2 blinks, you'll help them register for drivers' education classes!

Your reaction to the news that you have more than one baby on the way has most likely been a mix of strong emotions. I admit, the first month after discovering I was pregnant with twins, I probably looked like a deer caught in the headlights. A hundred questions ran through my mind. How could I be having twins? Is this really happening? How on earth can we handle 2 newborns at once?

You and your partner may be having very different reactions. While I was nervous, my husband was thrilled and breezily optimistic. He told me, "Relax, it will be great! Everything will work out just fine." I appreciated his joy and confidence, but I felt frustrated that he wasn't showing fear of the unknown, while I felt unsure of my ability to handle the situation. I wondered just how steep our learning curve would be to find our groove.

Here we are, years later, and we have not only survived but enjoyed the chaos and excitement of our twins' early years. I was so nervous when pregnant that I had imagined it would be more difficult than it actually was to raise newborn twins. In reality, the day-to-day routine of taking care of 2 little babies at the same time is very doable. Take things one step at a time, one day at a time. Once your family starts using some strategies to streamline your babies' care, you'll breathe more easily and enjoy the whole process.

The challenges of raising multiples are what make the parenting successes, and the overall experience, even sweeter. It is fascinating to watch as each child's unique personality evolves and develops over time. The highs and lows of the parenting experience are amplified for parents of multiples. You'll have moments of intense exhaustion but also moments of unsurpassed joy.

Have faith in yourself and your parenting abilities. The human spirit has an amazing ability to rise to a challenge. Any challenge in life must be tackled one step at a time, and parenting multiples is no exception. One particularly tough day may feel as if it lasts an eternity, but soon a time will come when you look back and wonder how the early weeks and months flew by so quickly.

## How to Handle More Than One Baby

You can care for twins or more by keeping in mind the basics of good parenting. A good parent provides love, safety, and security. When you look at the essentials, new babies need only a few things—something to eat (breast milk or formula), something to pee and poop into (diaper), a safe place to sleep (crib), and a safe way to ride in the car (car safety seat). If you streamline your ideas about what a newborn needs, remembering what is critical and what is optional, you can provide what is important to your newborns. Being able to tell the difference between basic requirements and the extras helps you stay organized and keep your sanity.

When you have baby twins, triplets, or more, an important mantra to remember is to *keep your babies on the same schedule.* Synchronizing schedules is a great way to happily survive the first year. When one baby wakes up to eat, wake up both babies for the feeding. If your babies' feedings are uncoordinated, you could easily spend the entire 24 hours of any given day feeding them, one after the other. If you feed 2 babies on 2 different schedules, you may not be able to sleep much, spend any time with an older child in your family, or recognize that vaguely familiar-looking person over there who reminds you of your partner.

---

### Parenting Support

Lisa, mom of twin toddlers, shares, "The best advice I got was to get and keep the babies on the same schedule. Managing the 2- to 3-hour bursts of handling the newborns' needs provides you some time to catch your breath when they are both sleeping, and it might possibly be the only shower opportunity one might have!"

---

## How Your Parenting Journey Changes

### The Early Years

Parenting multiples requires different skills at different stages. The earliest weeks and months with twins require stamina and an ability to streamline your daily tasks to survive with some semblance of sanity intact. As time wears on, you can ease out of survival mode and adjust to a different mind-set. You will be a master of understanding human emotions and interactions as you navigate all the different personalities that live under your roof. You will have as good of a grasp of interpersonal relations as an international diplomat.

### Pregnancy

During your pregnancy, channel your energy into preparing your nest for your babies. Twins and other multiples tend to deliver earlier than single-born babies, so prepare for this in case it happens (see the Preterm Birth and Other Birthing Challenges chapter on pages 211–224 for more information). Another reason you should prepare early is that your belly will get quite large and uncomfortable as you approach your due date. Start attending your local Parents of Multiples club meetings to meet other parents of multiples and start collecting helpful tips, and join online support groups. Pregnancy is also the time to enlist family and friends for help in the upcoming early weeks and months after your babies' birth.

> ## Parenting Support
> There is no one-size-fits-all parenting technique for raising multiples. Accept the advice of others, but do what works for *your* family.

## Early Infancy

During early infancy, your family will adjust quickly to a brand-new routine. The daily schedule will be filled with feedings, burpings, diaper changes, and catnaps, cycling through the days and nights. You and your infants will begin a relationship with each other that will strengthen with your love and consistent responses to their basic needs. You may discover during this period that while your infants were born at the same time, they have very different temperaments and personalities. Continue to show love and positive attention to older siblings in your family as well, and help them feel as much a part of the process as possible.

## Later Infancy

During later infancy, you'll coax everyone into a more predictable schedule, and your entire family will know what to expect at certain times. Your older babies are becoming little people, and you are beginning to see what makes each of them tick.

## The Toddler Years

When multiples are toddlers, life is overall much easier to handle, but you've got some major milestones ahead, such as toilet training and transitioning to big-kid beds. Strategies that work for single-born children need to be tweaked a bit when you're toilet training kids of the same age. All toddlers start to realize at some point that they are independent people, separate from their parents and their siblings. As a parent, help your toddlers make more decisions for themselves within an acceptable framework of behavior.

## The Preschool Years

The preschool years with multiples are such a great payoff for the years of effort. Your home evolves into their imagination factory. They sleep all night (for the most part!), they use the toilet to pee and poop (for the most part!), and you're now able to enjoy them even more and nurture each of them as unique people. One of the many benefits of having twins is that their "twinship" teaches them about patience and sharing; the multiples experience provides built-in life lessons. Many experts believe that multiples may be more socially savvy than their single-born peers because of the relationships they've grown with since infancy.

## The School Years and Beyond

In kindergarten and the school years, your multiples' world is rapidly expanding. As the years progress, keep in mind that parenting means raising future independent adults. You will make decisions about classroom placement, participation in activities, social dynamics, and more. Your children may already be quite independent, or you may be dealing with a fair amount of competition or interdependence between siblings.

# Enjoying Your Parenting Experience

Parenting multiples can be quite hectic, and in the early days and weeks, it can consume your days *and* nights. You don't want to merely *survive* raising them; you want to have fun, keep your sanity, and maintain good relationships with your partner and your other children. Mundane tasks must be done to keep the home running, in addition to our desire to create fun bonding experiences. Instead of folding laundry all day, it would be nice to cuddle with our kids and read them another good book. Most of us cannot afford to hire sitters or outside help regularly, and not all of us have family nearby who are able to help make our personal or couple time a routine experience.

As a parent of multiples, you'll need strategizing skills and creative planning to streamline and organize the everyday, necessary tasks as much as possible. That way, you have more time and energy to simply *be* with your kids. Another part of the equation of happy parenting is finding time for yourself, for your friends, to exercise, and to dedicate to your relationship with your partner.

Maintaining a routine household schedule will go a long way toward protecting special time for your multiples, your other children, yourself, and your partner. Your best ally during your twins' early years is their need for *sleep*. Young children need plenty of sleep. If your family works together to maintain a routine bedtime for your kids once they have grown past the newborn period, you will have a couple of hours free every night to spend with other family members or to think a complete sentence in your head without interruption! A happy parent is a better parent. It is not selfish to seek out personal or couple time. It is healthy and will have positive effects on everyone in your family. One cannot pour from an empty cup.

## One Size Does Not Fit All Families

My firsthand experiences taught me a lot as both a parent and a pediatrician. Our oldest son was only 18 months of age when our identical twin boys were born. My husband and I had to quickly figure out how to care for 3 kids, all younger than 2 years. I remember making a phone call to our crib manufacturer when we had a problem with one of our cribs. The woman helping me on the phone simply could not believe we had 3 kids in 3 cribs at the same time. *Efficiency* became our middle name as we coaxed ourselves and our 3 young sons to operate on a daily schedule so that we could all survive. We were both practicing physicians and had no outside child care assistance. My husband cared for our sons solo on the days that I worked in my pediatric practice, and I cared for them on his working days. Our fourth child, a daughter born a month before our oldest son turned 4 years of age, rounded out our family.

I continued to practice clinical pediatrics part-time through my twins' toddler years, and then I made the decision to stay home temporarily while my 4 children were young. Once all 4 kids were on a more regular school schedule, I returned to clinical practice and a university teaching faculty appointment. I can appreciate twin parenting from all angles—working outside the home, pumping breast milk, and working from home as your children's primary caregiver. My professional knowledge and real-life experience with 4 young kids has helped me learn strategies to efficiently, healthfully, and lovingly parent my children.

I appreciate the opportunity to share some of my insights with you and your family. Although this chapter and a few others in this book cover births of multiples in general, the following chapters, from preparing for your babies' arrival to the school years, focus on raising twins. However, all principals, strategies, tips, and advice mentioned throughout these chapters universally apply to families raising triplets, quadruplets, or more. For a specific chapter on triplets, quadruplets, and more, please see pages 225 to 232.

At times, friends, family, and health care professionals will be giving you advice and encouragement as you embark on *your* journey raising multiples. Listen to what everyone has to say and give ideas a try, but ultimately, only you can figure out what will work for your family and your situation. Not all families with multiples are the same. A family with 2 older kids and twins needs to operate much differently than a family of solely twin children or a family with triplets and one younger sibling. Accept the support and camaraderie of others, but *you* as the parent will find what works for your individual family. Have confidence in your own parenting judgment and abilities, and you will not only *survive* their early years but *enjoy* them.

# CHAPTER 2

# Preparing for Your Twins' Arrival

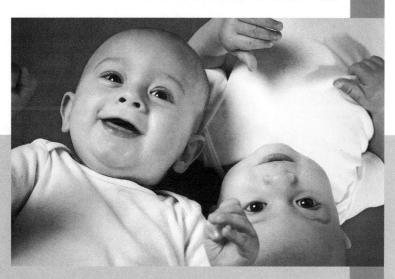

My husband and I always hoped to raise a big family. We were eager to get pregnant again soon after our first child was born. As a working mother, I figured I should be efficient and have kids as close in age as possible. (Pretty funny that it turned out to be minutes apart instead of years!) Happily, the result of our home pregnancy test soon turned positive, and at the 6-week mark I brought baby Matthew along to visit the obstetrician for what I thought would be a straightforward initial checkup.

I mentioned to my obstetrician that I had experienced some minimal bleeding yet was otherwise well. Apparently, the bleeding was enough to warrant an ultrasound.

I entered the small ultrasound room with Matthew in his stroller. The tiny room felt toasty warm from the large ultrasound machine and other running equipment. As we began, Matthew began to fuss, so I hoisted him onto the examination table with me and held him securely as I tried to position myself properly while lying flat on my back. Matthew was content when he saw how fun it was to swat at the examination table's crinkly paper. I continued to hold on to Matthew so that he wouldn't fall, no small feat during an uncomfortable vaginal ultrasound.

The ultrasound technician seemed to be taking quite a while. "Hmm... well, that's what I thought. OK, take a look at this," she said as she turned the monitor so that I could see it.

When you're looking at a fuzzy, moving, black-and-white image, it is challenging to interpret what you're seeing. But what I saw on that screen was unmistakable—2 tiny spots flickering repeatedly, each to its own rhythm. Two hearts! The world stopped as utter shock and disbelief filled every part of my mind. It felt as if I had stepped outside my body and was watching the scene play out, like watching a movie about someone, anyone, other than me. I plan everything—twins weren't part of my plan!

Through my dizzy blur of emotions, clutching onto a wriggling, oblivious Matthew, I kept focusing on those 2 blips on the screen. They were so beautiful, so innocent, sending their rhythmic beats across the sound waves like stars communicating in the Milky Way. I was mesmerized and terrified at the same time.

## Your Emotional Roller Coaster

The world of twins is an incredible, chaotic, remarkable, and challenging place. Unexpected joys will be yours as you watch your twins grow and develop relationships with each other and everyone in your family. Becoming a parent changes your life forever, but becoming a parent to multiples is truly a gift.

Like me, you will never forget the moment you learned you were pregnant with twins. Whether you conceived your babies naturally or with the assistance of fertility treatments, the reality that you are already the parent to more than one growing, living being is incredible. You may be very emotional about the news. Pregnancy, with all its associated hormones, is already an emotional time. That you'll have 2 (or more) bundles of joy, arriving at the same time, can increase the emotions. You may feel elated and joyous one moment, anxious and panicked the next. It doesn't matter whether your pregnancy was a surprise or planned for years; your emotional roller coaster is completely normal.

Your support network includes family and friends. These people know your history, and you may be able to share your deepest fears with them. Preserve your emotional well-being by discussing your feelings with your partner, your family, and your friends—anyone who is a good listener. Your excitement can transform into fear in mere moments, and discussions with loved ones is the best way to sort out your thoughts and begin to devise coping strategies. Make good use of your support network as a sounding board for what you are experiencing.

Along your new journey, you'll be developing new relationships as well. I suggest you reach out to your local Parents of Multiples club, at which you'll meet new families, in addition to registering for a multiples prenatal class at the hospital where you plan on delivering your babies. Even if you cannot attend in person regularly, it can be informative, as well as emotionally gratifying, to be surrounded by a room full of parents who are expecting or already have multiples.

You may feel alone and scared, but if you reach out, you will find other twin families who not only had a similar situation but also *survived* it and are richer people for having had the experience. Thanks to social media, if it's a challenge to physically attend Parents of Multiples club meetings in person, there are plenty of public and private groups online for support (read more in the Support, Emotional Health, and Time-savers chapter, specifically the Multiples of America section on pages 199–200). Online

### Twin Support

In the classic novel *The Hobbit* by J.R.R. Tolkien, the wizard Gandalf shows up on Bilbo Baggins' doorstep, informing him that he is to partake in a grand adventure involving dwarves, mountains, and a dragon. Bilbo, who loves the comfort of home and all that is familiar, is dumbfounded and incredulous. Parents of multiples may feel like Bilbo—that they have been nudged to begin an adventure into the unknown with little preamble, warning, or preparation.

support and other social media groups may be a necessity for you if you need bed rest during your pregnancy.

(For more information on finding a Parents of Multiples club near you, see the Support, Emotional Health, and Time-savers chapter, specifically pages 199–200.) You may find that your new friends who are pregnant with or already have twins or other multiples relate to your situation better than friends and family who you have known longer. It is comforting to talk with someone who is living a similar experience.

Ideally, the people you include in your support network should be positive and upbeat. Many well-meaning people may put their foot in their mouth when they learn that you are expecting multiples. These people might be as surprised and shocked as you were, when they learn the news. They may blurt poorly thought-out remarks or questions. In most cases, these people mean well and do not realize that they are being insensitive. Inconsiderate remarks may feel hurtful to you, especially in your state of emotional overdrive. Try not to let these comments get under your skin. The best way to respond is to simply say, "We are very surprised and happy." The nature of your children's conception isn't anyone else's business.

### Twin Support

You will likely have strangers asking you inappropriate questions such as about the conception of your twins or how much weight you have gained. Unfortunately, intrusive questions are not exclusive to those of us with multiples. I once read that Mary Kay Ash, founder of Mary Kay Cosmetics, was asked by a TV personality, "How old are you?" She looked her right in the eye and answered, "How much do you weigh?" Whether you respond with humor or sarcasm, don't let these interactions faze you. Respond concisely, or depending on the situation, simply ignore the question, and move forward.

Another option is to infuse humor. One mother I know had a standard response whenever anyone asked her, "What are you going to *do*?!" She would reply, "I'll just sell one of them on eBay!" The absurdity of this comment alerts questioners that they have asked an unhelpful and silly question. Regardless of how you choose to respond, don't be caught off guard; have your answer planned ahead of time so that you are prepared for this inevitable exchange. Most important, after your witty or concise reply, leave it at that. You don't need to get into details with the offender, and it will not help your emotional state to have this kind of conversation. If certain people in your life cannot be upbeat and supportive about your twin pregnancy, you may need emotional distance from those people for your sanity. Now is the time to take care of your body, your emotional status, and your babies.

 **Twin Support**

I met a woman right away at a Parent of Twins club meeting who was due to have her twins around her daughter's first birthday. I had been thinking I'd be the only mom in the country with 3 kids younger than 2 years, and suddenly here was a room full of people who could relate. Meeting these other parents diminished my feelings of isolation.

Many of us, consciously or not, may have imagined having a typical single-born baby and the way that single baby would fit into our lives and families. Allow yourself time to let go of any preconceived ideas you may have had. Learning that you will have more than one baby at the same time requires quite an adjustment of the mental picture of the future that we each create. Twins or more may not be what you expected or planned, but they have a way of providing you with happiness and love that you never thought possible.

When you feel overwhelmed or even nervous that you are expecting twins, feelings of guilt may not be far behind. You may think, "All my friends have it so easy, having only one baby at a time. It would be so much easier to give birth to just *one* baby than to have twins. But I shouldn't feel this way. How can I feel this way when I am so lucky to be having twins?" Allow yourself to feel the full range of human emotions, and let go of the guilt. If you feel disappointed at times, acknowledge your feelings and then move forward. Use this time to talk with your partner and supportive friends.

**Twin Tale**

Jon, dad to infant twins and a preschool-aged singleton, shares, "I wish I knew how elastic the human capacity for love and care truly is. My worry that we wouldn't be able to deftly handle all of the intricacies of [baby] care times 2, *and* still find time to soak up all the love and wonder without going crazy, quickly gave way to a rhythm that—almost as quickly as it fell upon us—became the 'new normal.' We can't even imagine *only* having one baby."

# Taking Care of Your Body and Pregnancy

That you are carrying more than one baby places you into a special category in the eyes of obstetricians. A pregnancy with twins is classified as a *high-risk* pregnancy, which can be translated simply as "We need to monitor this pregnancy more closely." Most twin pregnancies progress smoothly, and the odds of a healthy pregnancy increase if you take better care of yourself.

When doctors discuss the length of time a baby was growing before birth, they call it *gestation* and use weeks and days to define it. For example, a doctor may say that a baby was born at 36³/₇ weeks' gestation. This means that the baby was growing for 36 weeks and 3 days.

According to the National Vital Statistics Reports, about 60% of twins, more than 90% of triplets, and virtually all quadruplets and higher-order multiples are born preterm. Most single-baby pregnancies last an average of 39 weeks; for twins, 35 weeks; for triplets, 32 weeks; and for quadruplets, 29 weeks. The length of pregnancy decreases with each additional baby.

The American College of Obstetricians and Gynecologists defines *preterm* deliveries as those occurring on or before 36⁶/₇ weeks' gestation, *early-term* babies as those born 37⁰/₇ weeks of gestation through 38⁶/₇ weeks of gestation, and *full-term* as 39⁰/₇ weeks of gestation through 40⁶/₇ weeks of gestation. Parents who are expecting twins or more should be aware of the greater likelihood of preterm deliveries. Please note that *early term* is distinctive from *preterm*. For more information on preterm delivery, please refer to the Preterm Birth and Other Birthing Challenges chapter on pages 211 to 224.

Proper nutrition is a very important consideration during your pregnancy. Pregnant mothers should take a prenatal vitamin with folic acid, ideally starting a few months ahead of when they hope to conceive, if possible. Folic acid, an important ingredient in prenatal vitamins, has definitively been proven to reduce the chances of neural tube defects such as spina bifida. If you haven't started taking a prenatal vitamin daily yet, don't fret about the missed time, but do start now. Take your prenatal vitamin with food to reduce nausea, and applaud yourself for taking yet another step to keep your babies as healthy as possible. Moms of twins don't need 2 prenatal vitamins a day—one is enough.

Eating the proper foods and the right amount of calories is critical during a twin pregnancy. Whereas single-baby pregnancies require 300 extra calories a day, most experts agree that twin pregnancies require around 1,000 extra calories a day. Morning sickness can be eased by eating small, healthy snacks frequently and can help you reach your caloric goals each day. Keeping a little something in your stomach at all times can help take the edge off the nausea. Yogurt, nuts, fruit, smoothies, crackers, and protein shakes are all good options.

In addition to consuming extra calories, drinking water throughout the day is important. Keeping well hydrated may drive you crazy in later months when it seems as if you're running to the bathroom every 5 minutes; however, your babies' blood flow and removal of wastes depends on it. It may help to drink more water earlier in the day and then stop after 8:00 pm so that you can sleep longer stretches at night between bathroom breaks.

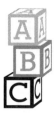

### Twin Tip

Every morning, pre-fill your daily water needs in individual water bottles or a bigger container. Take sips of water every hour. At the end of the day, empty bottles will tell you that you drank what you needed.

## Listening to Your Body's Signs

Regular prenatal visits with the obstetric team are vital. Because twins have an increased chance of being born early, any symptoms or concerns *must* be addressed in a timely fashion for the safety of your babies. Any new pregnancy symptoms you notice *should* be brought to your obstetrician's attention. Seemingly minor things could be a sign of something more serious. Bleeding or vaginal discharge, contractions that are becoming more frequent, pressure in the pelvis or lower back, or even diarrhea can all be signs of preterm labor. And while early bleeding in the first trimester could be the normal phenomenon of your twins implanting into the uterine wall, you should call your obstetrician if you experience bleeding at any point.

 **Twin Tale**

Lisa, mom to toddler twins, shares, "I think that anyone expecting multiples should get a lot more information about what to expect in the event of a C-section. Looking back, I wish I'd been a little more prepared for it."

Twin pregnancies can also increase the chance of preeclampsia, a condition during which a mother has increased blood pressure, protein in the urine (detectable by urinalysis, which is why every prenatal visit necessitates a urine sample), and more swelling than is normal during pregnancy. If you notice rapid weight gain or new headaches, alert your obstetrician so that you may be examined as soon as possible. Depending on the severity of the situation, treatment may range from bed rest, to hospital-administered medications, to the necessary delivery of your babies.

*Twin-to-twin transfusion syndrome, or TTTS,* is a rare occurrence for identical twins (10%–20% of monochorionic twin pregnancies, meaning identical twins who share one placenta). The 2 babies' blood can mix in a connection between placental vessels, resulting in one baby receiving too much blood, while the other baby receives too little. Prenatal ultrasounds can allow obstetricians to study the placenta, blood flow, and growth and development of identical twins.

An optimistic yet attentive attitude during your pregnancy will help your mental state during this important time. Take things one day at a time and one week at a time. Eat well and pay attention to what your body and your babies are telling you. Every extra day that your babies spend inside the womb will help them once delivery day arrives. The bigger your belly gets, the bigger your smile should be!

## Pregnancy Preparations

The more you do now to prepare for twins will help immensely once your babies arrive. If you are on a form of bed rest because of pregnancy complications, you will need to delegate preparation tasks or order supplies online as much as possible. Consider obtaining necessary items, such as cribs, a bit earlier in the pregnancy than you would for a traditional single-baby pregnancy, so that you're ready in case your babies decide to show up early.

## New Information on Parenting Twins

Parents of Multiples clubs, whether online or in person, can offer emotional support and provide useful information. Even 1 or 2 useful tips may really help you out logistically with twin babies, saving you hours of time and effort down the line. I learned at a Parents of Twins club meeting about the existence of a twin-feeding pillow, a large foam-filled device specially designed to make it easy to breastfeed or bottle-feed both babies simultaneously. I had never heard of it before, even though I was a pediatrician! This single tip made our family's lives incredibly easier during those first few months. I cannot imagine surviving those early weeks without my trusty twin-feeding pillow.

## Bargain Shopping for Twins

Parents of Twins clubs also host clothing and equipment swaps and sales of gently used items from other members. Real bargains can be found at these sales. Kids grow incredibly fast and need new clothes seemingly every week, so these bargains can be helpful for your budget.

You must shop carefully when preparing your nest for twins. The baby product industry would have you believe that you need 20 pairs of baby booties for each baby, a dust ruffle for each crib, a baby wipe warmer, and a diaper pail for every room in the house. Advertisers even go insofar as to publish "handy" checklists with many unnecessary or irrelevant items. Feel free to use these lists as reminders or guides, but don't feel obligated to buy all the items on them.

First-time parents especially need to be aware of the baby product marketing phenomenon. Because they are your first babies, you want to prepare as best you can. Baby product companies take advantage of new parents' feelings of anticipation, anxiety, and inexperience by subtly hinting that if you are to be a good parent, you'll definitely purchase the crib mobile with the alphabet on it for just $49.99. However, expensive things are *not* what make you a good parent. A good parent provides love, safety, and security. All the other things are just bells and whistles.

Parents of twins need to make budgeting a priority. You have to buy or launder twice as many diapers, and you need twice the bottle supplies if you

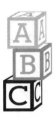

**Twin Tip**

Is your head spinning over too many "must-have" baby items? Many baby products are unnecessary. As long as you have the basics, such as food, diapers, cribs, clothes, and car safety seats, you're set.

are pumping or not breastfeeding. Consider membership to a bulk warehouse store to save on needed supplies.

You will probably need to streamline other areas that are negotiable. Over the long haul, however, twins are not much more expensive than 2 babies born separately. It's just that you will need certain things at the same time.

Reach out to your extended family and friends, and ask whether they have any baby items they don't need anymore. Borrowing is wonderful because a lot of baby gear is useful for only a few months. Bouncy seats, carriers, and baby swings are quickly outgrown. For example, a soft front-pack carrier can start to be used when a baby is around 8 pounds (check the specific manufacturer's instructions) and continue to be used until the baby is up to around 20 pounds, which is usually by 9 months of age. Don't be overly particular about hand-me-downs. I remember during my first pregnancy, I wanted to buy everything new and fresh for my son. Months later, cycling through different stages so quickly, I realized, "Hey, it really isn't a big deal to borrow a baby swing and save some cash."

Make sure you carefully examine and clean borrowed equipment to ensure that it is safe. Verify that it has no loose or broken parts. When you borrow items, you also need to make sure they are not on any safety recall listings. Check the US Consumer Product Safety Commission website at www.cpsc.gov to make sure your borrowed items have not been recalled. This is especially important for cribs because your twins will spend most of their first months there.

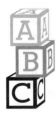

**Twin Tip**

When preparing your nest for twins, stay on a budget by borrowing extra baby equipment. But make sure that borrowed or secondhand baby gear has not been recalled by checking the US Consumer Product Safety Commission website (www.cpsc.gov).

Other "must-have" baby items are usually unnecessary or even unsafe. You'll have to decide for yourself whether certain items are worth buying to have a cute nursery or you'd rather save the money. Other items may be unnecessary. A good example is a crib bumper. The American Academy of Pediatrics recommends not using one at all. Crib bumpers (or bumper pads) may seem as though they can help protect babies from drafts and bumps, but they should not be used in cribs. There is no evidence that bumper pads can prevent serious injuries; in fact, they pose a risk of suffocation, strangulation, or entrapment. In addition, older babies can use them for climbing out of the crib. Babies usually do not roll over for the first 3 or 4 months, so you don't need to worry about them hitting their heads on the rails. Evaluate so-called necessary baby items to ensure that they are needed or even safe.

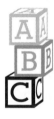

**Twin Tip**

I cannot stress this enough: babies require your love and hugs more than stuff or cute outfits.

# Twin Baby Gear: What You Need

Here is a list of items your babies will need, along with items that you may not need but *will* save your sanity. Though the list is not all-inclusive, it provides items to consider purchasing for the early months of twin baby parenting. Items that are useful later in your twins' lives are discussed in subsequent chapters.

- **Cribs.** Your twins will sleep safely and comfortably in separate cribs. Buy either 2 new cribs or just one if an older sibling has outgrown his or her crib that meets current safety standards. (Check www.cpsc. gov for the most up-to-date recall information.) If a trusted friend or family member has an extra crib you can use, great, but do your homework and make sure the crib is not broken or on a safety recall list. A crib's slats should be no wider than 2⅜ inches. The top of the crib rail should be at least 26 inches from the top of the mattress. (Periodically lower the mattress as your children get taller.) Implemented in 2011, federal safety standards prohibit the manufacture or sale of drop-side rail cribs to prevent suffocation or strangulation that leads to newborn and infant deaths.

- **Car safety seats.** You definitely need 2 of these. A car safety seat is the one item (or should I say 2 items?) you should not borrow or take as a hand-me-down. If a car safety seat has been involved in even a minor crash, it must be replaced. Car safety seats have a Lower Anchors and Tethers for Children (LATCH) system that makes proper installation much easier for a car that is LATCH ready. (This system became standard in 2002.) You can install your car safety seats by LATCH or by seat belts; make sure you read your specific car owner's manual carefully for instructions, as well as the instructions that come with the car safety seats. Because twins are small at birth, you'll need a *newborn/infant* car safety seat, preferably with head and neck support. Don't worry about convertible car safety seats until later, as your newborns will probably not be the designated minimum weight at birth. (For more information on newborn/infant car safety seats, visit HealthyChildren.org.)

- **Breast milk or formula.** Ideally, your babies' food will be breast milk in the beginning weeks, but you may want or need to use newborn/infant formula to supplement breastfeeding or feed exclusively. We discuss breast milk and formula-feeding issues at much greater length in the next 2 chapters.

- **Bottles, nipple rings, and silicone nipples.** You'll find that a dishwasher will make cleaning feeding items much easier. The sanitize settings on most modern dishwashers will effectively sterilize your equipment for you. Small plastic dishwashing baskets (available online or in the baby section of any big-box store) can hold the nipples and nipple rings in place during a dishwashing cycle. Also, make sure that you have newborn slow-flow nipples on hand (there are medium- and fast-flow options for when your twins have grown). Newborns typically feed on breast milk 8 to 12 times in 24 hours (on formula, a little less frequently), so you should estimate your needs and know that you may need as many as 24 nipples in 24 hours. You could make a choice to have less, but then you'll need to sanitize the used nipples several times throughout the day. If you'll be using a breast pump, make sure your bottle supplies are compatible with the pump.

- **Breast pump.** A pump is infinitely useful if you plan on breastfeeding your twins. If you find that you need to boost your milk supply, pumping will help stimulate your breasts to produce more milk, and you can store your nutritious milk for a later feeding. A high-quality electric double breast pump will be worth the investment when it saves you time and energy collecting breast milk. Many moms choose to rent a breast pump rather than buy one up front; rentals allow parents a little more flexibility in the budget. Breastfeeding twins is discussed in much further detail in the next 2 chapters.

- **Diapers and wipes.** Disposable diapers are quite convenient but expensive. Log on to major diaper manufacturers' websites to obtain coupons for parents of multiples. You may need to wait until you have birth certificates because some companies want proof that you actually have twins. Many families use cloth diapers and launder them themselves or use a cloth diaper service. The cost and availability of these services vary from region to region, so you will need to do some investigation. Cloth diapers can be more environmentally friendly than disposables that fill up landfills, but on the other hand, cloth diapers require more energy and water use for all the washings. Be aware that even sensitive-skin wipes may irritate your babies' skin, so hold off on buying a lot until you're sure you've got a good match. My own kids' skin was quite sensitive so often we used warm water and cotton balls to prevent diaper rashes (for more on diaper rash, please see the Early Infancy and Getting on a Schedule chapter, specifically the Diaper Rash section on pages 72–73).

- **Twin-feeding pillow.** Before you are 6 months' pregnant, obtain a twin-feeding pillow so that you are ready in case your twins deliver early. The twin-feeding pillow is a wonderfully simple invention that makes simultaneous feedings much easier. It is helpful for either breastfeeding or bottle-feeding 2 babies at the same time. I used mine from the time my twins were born to about when they were 7 or 8 months of age. Feeding your babies simultaneously saves time and helps keep your twins on the same daily schedule.

- **Changing table.** Once you have changed a few diapers while slouching over the bed or the floor, you'll realize that the health and comfort of your back may depend on a changing table. Even if you have a safety strap on the changing pad, *never* step away from the table, even for a moment. Even a newborn can wiggle her way off the table if you are not there holding a hand on her. Our family mounted a changing pad on a dresser upstairs so that we could have one changing area upstairs and one downstairs. A second changing table is not a necessity, but it sure made life easier for those first few months.

- **Clothing.** Do you prefer to let laundry pile up and deal with it once a week? Or do you prefer to launder more manageable piles more frequently? Your answer to these laundry questions will help you decide how much clothing to obtain for your twins. For clothes to wear at home, no one cares whether your twins stay in pajamas all day. You may need 2 or 3 outfits a day per twin depending on spit-ups and overflowed diapers. Babies grow fast, so don't buy too many newborn-sized clothes—these may be outgrown quickly. Important clothing and layette items include

  - All-in-one shirts that snap closed at the crotch, as well as separate tops and bottoms
  - Socks (Shoes are not needed until your babies are walking.)
  - "Swaddle sacks" for ease in safely swaddling your babies
  - Footed pajama sets
  - Sack-like pajamas with an open bottom hem to simplify overnight diaper changes
  - Receiving blankets for swaddling
  - Baby washcloths and hooded towels for bath time

- **Newborn/infant washtub for bathing.** One should suffice, as before your babies are able to sit independently, the safest way to bathe them is one after the other. Once your babies are able to sit independently (see the Later Infancy and First Birthday chapter, specifically the second "Twin Tip" on page 91), you'll be able to bathe them simultaneously in a regular bathtub, always with constant supervision and within arm's reach.

- **Twin stroller.** There is a range of prices and styles for twin strollers. A tandem front-back stroller is more convenient for younger babies because you can often snap the newborn/infant car safety seats right into it. This type of stroller is also narrower and thus easier to get through doorways for your pediatrician visits (which are more frequent in the first months). Side-by-side strollers are nicer for older babies and toddlers because your twins can interact more in this style. They are wider than the tandem front-back strollers and do not fit through standard doorways, but they usually fit through doorways wide enough for a wheelchair. The more expensive options can be quite lightweight, so if you live in a city and use your stroller every day, you may want to make this investment. Be sure to check the stroller's baby weight minimum and maximum rules to be sure your babies will be safe in the stroller.

- **Waterproof mattress pads to protect crib mattresses.** In addition, smaller waterproof pads placed on top of the crib sheets makes cleaning after spit-ups or other spills much easier. You simply take away the soiled pad and replace it with a fresh pad, saving the time of remaking an entire crib with new sheets.

- **Front-pack carrier, wrap, or sling.** These carriers have a limited life span but can make your life easier when trying to get things done around the house. A second carrier means your partner can carry your other twin. Baby slings are another great option. As with all baby equipment, ensure that your sling meets current safety standards and that you are using it properly to reduce suffocation risks.

- **Play yard(s).** These are useful for keeping your babies safe in different areas of your home when you need to answer the phone or run to the bathroom. Some models come with a changing table attachment so that you can have a diaper changing station in your main family area; extra diapers, wipes, and burp cloths can be stored in the lower compartment. When choosing to use this, do not add a supplemental mattress or any other padding to the play yard.

- **A good camera (or a smartphone with a camera).** With twins, you'll take countless pictures, but only a small proportion of all shots taken may be photoprint worthy. Thankfully, smartphones usually come with

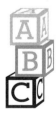

## Twin Tip

Take plenty of pictures of each of your twins *alone,* as well as together. They will thank you later for treating them as individuals. How can you remember who is who in the pictures? Color-coding their clothes will help you identify them years later, if you aren't able to label the photos in a timely fashion. Boys and girls lend themselves to different color codes pretty easily. Alternatively, one twin can wear primarily solid colors, while your other wears prints or stripes.

a terrific digital camera that also takes great videos. Be sure to back up your photos to an online cloud or an external hard drive. I admit, I fell behind quickly on logging our digital images into printed photo books. However, I am hoping that my stored digital images will find fresh light with future technology.

- **Diaper pail with deodorizer system.** Diaper pails trap odors with varying degrees of success and usually require daily disposal to eliminate odors. Breast milk stools don't have much of a foul odor, so if you are breastfeeding, a diaper pail may be unnecessary. In my experience, when solid foods are started at around 6 months of age, the diapers start to emit a stronger odor that even the best pail can't cover. Our family found it easiest to store dirty diapers in an ordinary lined trash can kept inside the garage, away from our noses.

- **Rocking chair or glider.** Once your twins are strong enough, they can sit on your lap with support while the 3 of you read a book together. This is especially nice as part of your nighttime routine to help signal to your babies that it will soon be time to sleep. In the early months, you will probably need help in picking up your twins when you have finished reading, but you'll find yourself becoming more self-sufficient with such tasks as time progresses and your babies' muscle tone strengthens.

- **Bulletin board or comparable organizational system.** It is important (particularly if your babies were born early or small) to keep track of baby feedings and soiled diapers, and record keeping can quickly become overwhelming. Have a system for recording your babies' feedings, wet diapers, and poopy diapers in a central location of your home.

## Twin Preparation Checklist

- Two cribs
- Two car safety seats
- Breast milk or formula
- Bottles, nipple rings, and silicone nipples
- Breast pump
- Diapers and wipes
- Twin-feeding pillow
- Changing table
- Clothing
- Newborn/infant washtub for bathing
- Twin stroller
- Waterproof mattress pads
- Front-pack carrier, wrap, or sling
- Play yard(s)
- Camera
- Diaper pail with deodorizer system
- Rocking chair or glider
- Bulletin board or comparable organizational system

you weren't already an organized person, don't worry. Parents of multiples become quite organized very quickly to keep up with everybody's needs. Smartphone apps can also come in handy for recording breast-feeding and soiled diaper data, but you may prefer an old-fashioned board or notebook as a centralized method of record keeping so that multiple caregivers can consult and make notes on it.

## Preparing Older Siblings

The arrival of a new baby creates a whole new family environment and requires adjustment on behalf of all family members. With the arrival of twins, the family dynamic changes even more dramatically. Older siblings' lives will invariably change with the arrival of 2 or more newborns who rely on their parents to take care of all their needs. The proper way to prepare your older children for your twin birth depends on their ages and developmental levels.

**Twin Support**

When preparing older siblings for the birth of twins, books are a terrific resource. Age-appropriate books are an excellent way to help a child of any age through a multitude of transitions.

In the first trimester before the pregnancy begins to show, you may want to hold off on explanations to children younger than 3. A good time to periodically talk about the arrival of new babies is after the pregnancy has progressed 12 weeks and you are starting to show. Toddlers especially enjoy picture books of babies, and age-appropriate baby doll sets are a fun way to pretend play before your babies' arrival. Keep in mind that it will be difficult for your child to imagine life with your twins until it actually happens.

Once your twins arrive and come home, they will mainly require feeding, changing, and snuggling. All this can be accomplished while you engage your older child in conversation and play. Your twins' language development will benefit from observing you and their older siblings chat. Let your twins relax in their bouncy chairs and watch while, for example, you and their big sister work on a craft project together.

**Twin Tale**

Jon, dad to infant twins plus an older son, says, "I wish I'd been more prepared to introduce my firstborn (singleton) to his siblings. I was a nervous wreck. 'Will we still be best buds? Will I be able to devote to him anything close to the attention he received before [my] twins arrived?' He was fine, of course, and immediately fell in love with his sisters."

Try to avoid major lifestyle changes for older siblings around the time that your twins are born. Becoming a big sibling is enough of a lifestyle transition for a young child already. Now is not the time to move your older child to a big-kid bed, for example. If a room trade must be made for space issues, make the trade earlier in the pregnancy so that your child does not feel he has been replaced by your twins. If your older child has been toilet-trained, you might expect some toileting accidents (wetting or soiling). Regressive behaviors during the adjustment period are normal and common as a child adjusts to life with new siblings in his family. You will have a lot on your plate caring for 2 new babies, and you might find yourself frustrated if your older child is acting out as a call for attention. Be as understanding of your older child as you can be, as challenging as that may be, given all your new responsibilities.

If your child will be younger than 2 years when your twins are born, you will deal with fewer sibling rivalry issues. Toddlers younger than 2 are much more adaptable and seem to take the birth of a new baby more in stride. The greatest challenge is for a child 2 to 3 years of age. As an older child, he has a better understanding of what is going on yet still craves lots of love and attention from his parents, as any child does.

If sibling rivalry issues take hold, make sure to make time for one-on-one attention with your older child. He can go shopping with just you or have bath time with just your partner. Daily special time together, apart from your babies, will go a long way to reassure your older child that he'll always be loved. Even if you don't have child care available for your twins so that you can take your older child on an outing, you can use your babies' nap times for special one-on-one time with your older child. Newborns sleep most of the 24 hours in a day, so this will allow more time to spend with your other child than you may think. Of course, the big challenge, which is discussed at length in the next 2 chapters, is to help your twins sleep *at the same time* so that everyone can live a healthier, calmer, less chaotic life.

# Nearing Your Delivery

As you advance through pregnancy and prepare for your babies' big arrival, your belly will expand as you've never thought possible. As challenging as carrying 2 babies can be, savor each day of your pregnancy. Every day in the womb is so critical for your babies' development. Applaud yourself for eating well and keeping them healthy. Pack your hospital bag early, get lots of rest, and put your feet up at every opportunity.

Check with your obstetric team regarding your hospital options for delivery, and refer to the Preterm Birth and Other Birthing Challenges chapter on pages 211 to 224. Be mentally prepared for the fact that a twin delivery means a lot of extra people in the room with you. More personnel and nursing is required to ensure the safety of and provide necessary measures for your babies upon delivery.

I delivered my twins in a university hospital setting via cesarean delivery, so with my own obstetric team, the neonatal intensive care unit teams, and various attendings, residents, and interns, it made for quite the crowd. When a friend of mine delivered quadruplets, her hospital used 2 operating rooms so that there was enough space for the delivery team and proper support for the immediate care of her 4 babies. No matter how prepared you feel for the delivery, the reality of it will be quite an adventure. *Your* delivery experience will be uniquely yours and yours alone.

# CHAPTER 3

# The Early Days and Weeks

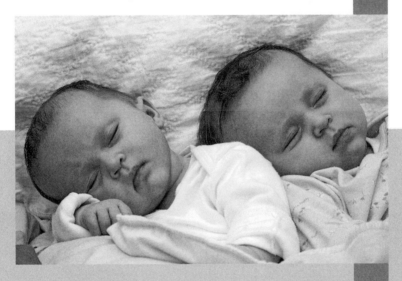

*W*hen your delivery day finally arrives, you may feel a mixture of relief and trepidation. The months of wondering what the deliveries would be like and *when* the deliveries would happen, and perhaps some time on bed rest, are all now at an end. One chapter is closing, while a new chapter begins.

## In the Hospital

Your babies may be born full-term, or they may deliver preterm. In either case, rely on your hospital's medical staff for guidance and advice. Neonatal intensive care unit (NICU) nurses, NICU physicians, and other newborn nursery staff members, such as respiratory therapists and dietitians, bring a wealth of experience and knowledge to the table. Avail yourself of the hospital staff's medical and practical advice at every opportunity. The NICU and newborn nurses have seen it all. There is no such thing as a silly question, especially if you are a first-time parent. Better to ask and have your questions resolved than to fret quietly about a concern that may be typical for newborns.

If possible, arrange for assistance at home ahead of time to care for your older children, which will allow both parents to be present and working together during the hospital stay. Having both partners at the hospital helps you recover more smoothly from the deliveries. In addition, a teamwork approach then begins from day 1, which helps align expectations so that all caregivers stay on the same page moving forward.

 **Twin Tale**

Mike, dad to school-aged twins, recalls, "Even though we had an older child, and although we felt prepared for the experience, our hospital stay felt surreal—this [was] really happening!"

Don't feel guilty if you employ the help of the overnight nursing staff to care for your newborn twins so that you can get some nighttime sleep, physically recover from the births, and prepare for your homecoming. You shouldn't feel that you have to do it all while you are in the hospital. You are still recovering from the births yourself, and if you cannot recover properly, you will not be able to care for anyone else. Think of the emergency procedures on an airplane: first you must put your own oxygen mask on, and then you can help others with their oxygen masks. You cannot effectively care for your babies if you are not operational yourself. There will be plenty of time for you to do it all when you are back home with your babies. Very quickly you will be home, wishing you had someone to ask whether your babies' poop looks normal or what good burping positions to try.

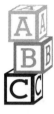

### Twin Tip

Ask plenty of questions when you are in the hospital. With all the excitement, labor, and sleep deprivation, you may forget your important questions as they pop into your mind, so keep a pen and notepad or your smartphone by your bedside to jot down thoughts for when your pediatrician and nurses are making rounds and checking in with your family.

While you are in the hospital, the newborn nursery nurses can show you good techniques to swaddle a newborn, an important lesson for first-time parents, which helps soothe a fussy newborn or infant by mimicking the close womb environment. Even seasoned parents can use a refresher course in good swaddling techniques. For more information on swaddling, visit HealthyChildren.org/swaddling.

Lactation consultants can help you with the breastfeeding process. Ensure that your pediatrician or registered nurse (also known as an RN) requests a lactation consultation on your behalf if the hospital doesn't automatically provide one for you. The lactation consultant can help your new babies figure out how to latch on correctly, show you different ways to tandem feed your twins simultaneously, and show you how to pump and store your breast milk. The NICU nurses can also help you learn how to administer medications, if your babies will need them.

### Twin Support

Parents have a greater chance of breastfeeding success by educating themselves ahead of time with strong breastfeeding resources. Two excellent references to have on hand are the American Academy of Pediatrics *New Mother's Guide to Breastfeeding* edited by Joan Younger Meek, MD, MS, RD, FAAP, FABM, IBCLC, and *The Nursing Mother's Companion* by Kathleen Huggins. Also refer to the Breastfeeding Twins: How to Do It section on pages 42 to 44.

All too soon, you will find yourself loading your babies into their car safety seats, discharge papers in your hand, with the all clear to take your babies home on their first voyages outside the womb and the hospital.

## Coming Home

Bringing your newborn twins home from the hospital can be a relief. Returning to your familiar, comfortable home, bed, and nonhospital food feels good. But then the realization hits—you have 2 little babies to take care of! Where are the helpful nurses and hospital staff with their extra hands? Take a deep breath and take things one day at a time. Your babies will get stronger and bigger every day, and your family will learn a new way of living, your new normal, so to speak, that includes your new babies. Think of life with your twins as a great sailing adventure on the high seas. Your homecoming is when you start to learn to tie knots and hoist the sails. You're just hitting the waters now, and soon you'll achieve a cruising speed and be sailing on an incredible journey.

If your twins have older siblings, now is a great time to celebrate *them* and to view your twins' arrival from their point of view as well. I recommend discussing your new babies in as positive of terms as possible with your other child(ren). For example, "Here are your new little sisters. How fortunate they are to have you as a big sister!" Lavish as much attention as you can on your older child. Your babies have no idea whether you're talking to them anyway, but your older child does. You'd be amazed at the great conversations you can have with an older child while you are burping your twins. Extend this philosophy to others. When well-meaning relatives and friends visit to coo over your adorable newborns, remind them ahead of time to please say hello to your older children first and to include them in the conversation as much as possible.

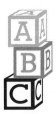

### Twin Tip

Your twins' birth means that your older children are now big siblings. Some families like to highlight older kids' new titles by giving them big-sibling gifts from the new twins to celebrate their new family status.

# Keeping Twins on the Same Schedule: Starting Now

How will you manage and survive your babies' first weeks after birth? Well, the good news is that newborns sleep *a lot.* Eating and sleeping are the 2 main concerns of any newborn. The key to *your* survival is to use this to your advantage and make sure that your twins start sleeping at similar times. On average, newborns need 16 or 17 hours of sleep in a 24-hour day. Inconveniently, their sleep is evenly divided between daytime and nighttime, with frequent interruptions for feeding. All newborns need to eat at least every 3 hours because their stomachs are so small, yet their caloric needs are great. Breastfed newborns may need to eat every 1 to 2 hours in occasional cluster feeding. Frequent breastfeeding sessions help boost your milk supply and accommodate your child's growth spurts.

So how do you coordinate the chaos of 2 babies needing to eat and sleep in such frequent spurts? Here is the golden rule for feeding twins: *when one wakes up to eat, both must wake up to eat.* Despite the old saying "Never wake a sleeping baby," remember that you will not have enough hours in a day to feed one after the other is fed, day in, day out. Once your babies are awake to eat, feed them at the same time, with burping breaks throughout and a good burping session at the end. If you have a helping hand to feed one twin while you feed your other, great. But if you are breastfeeding, or ever plan on being alone with your twins, you'll need to teach yourself how to feed both babies simultaneously. Both moms *and* dads might as well start learning how to feed their babies simultaneously together early on, while support from the recent deliveries is still available.

 **Twin Tale**

Sheri, mom to preschool-aged twins, recalls, "The best advice I received was to feed the babies at the same time. Never would have thought of that on my own."

The best way to feed both twins simultaneously is with a large twin-feeding pillow, which works for breastfeeding and bottle-feeding (Figures 3-1 and 3-2). It is a large U-shaped pillow with a firm foam core that fits around your waist and the opening at your back. Most versions have a safety belt to latch into place so that the pillow remains snug to your body. Each twin gets his or her own side and feeds in the football hold position. You will likely need help positioning your babies on the pillow in the early days, but you will learn how to position them by yourself with time. You will soon be very capable, handling both babies safely simultaneously.

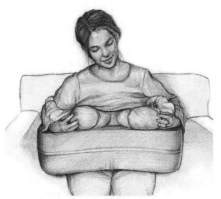

**Figure 3-1.** Double football hold position for breastfeeding.

If you've had a cesarean delivery, you may need to wait a week or so before starting to use a twin-feeding pillow because the pillow's front edge crosses your healing abdomen. In the postoperative period, use bed pillows propped on both sides to breastfeed your twins in a double football hold position. An alternative breastfeeding position has one baby in the traditional cradle hold and one baby in the football hold (Figure 3-3). Fathers can jump right in with tandem feeding their babies, using the specialized

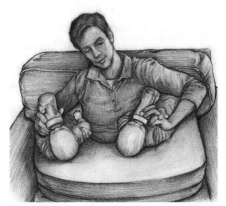

**Figure 3-2.** Double football hold position for bottle-feeding.

pillow, with bottles filled with pumped breast milk or formula.

Positioning standard bed pillows or throw pillows for each feeding is a nuisance because you must get the right fit each time for the frequent newborn feedings. Position yourself and your twins properly for feedings, whether breastfeeding or bottle-feeding, to prevent backaches from poor posture. Hunching over for 20 minutes at a time, 8 to 12 times a day, can take a toll on the body after a few weeks.

Twins, especially if born early, have very small stomachs yet large caloric needs. This is why new babies need to feed frequently, both day and night, to properly grow and gain weight in these critical early weeks after birth. One possible newborn feeding schedule is outlined in the next 3 paragraphs. Feel free to tailor this schedule to your own babies' needs.

When your twins wake up to eat, look at the clock and make a mental note of the time. Newborns often can tolerate being awake for only an hour or an hour and a half at a stretch, 2 hours tops. That they can be awake only roughly 90 minutes at a time can help you adjust your twins to live on the same schedule. How is the

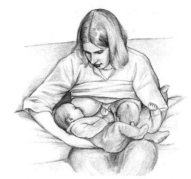

**Figure 3-3.** Alternative breastfeeding position with one baby in traditional cradle hold and one baby in football hold.

time awake spent? Feeding and burping will take quite some time (especially as parents work on positioning their babies correctly). After feeding and burping, your twins should get some time upright to help them digest their milk. This is a nice time to interact, talk, and play with them. Bouncy chairs are helpful to keep one baby upright, safely buckled in, while you cuddle or burp your other twin.

After a feeding is an ideal pooping time for babies because of the *gastrocolic reflex,* when food in the stomach stimulates the bowels to move. If you wait a bit after feeding to change diapers, you may save money on diapers by anticipating the stool in advance. After all the action of feeding, burping, and diaper changing, take another look at the clock. I can assure you it is probably almost time for your twins to go back to sleep. They may not appear particularly fussy, but remember that crying is a late indicator of fatigue. Don't wait for a newborn to cry to put her down to sleep. Once she is crying, the adrenaline has kicked in, and she will be overly agitated and

 **Twin Tale**

While we were in the hospital after Andrew and Ryan's birth, I was worried about Ryan. It was always Andrew who awoke for the next feeding, and we found ourselves waking Ryan up with virtually every feeding to stay coordinated with Andrew's schedule. He gained weight just fine in those early weeks, despite always being woken sooner than he seemed ready for feedings. All these years later, Ryan has proven himself to have a calm, cool, and collected personality, laid-back and relaxed. I am convinced he illustrated these same characteristics to us as a days-old newborn.

stimulated, making it *more* difficult for her to settle to sleep. You will learn to identify your babies' subtler clues that they are ready to nap, ahead of the point of no return. Swaddle your twins in swaddling or receiving blankets to mimic the womb environment. At this point, they are fed, burped, and have a clean diaper, so they have nothing left on their agenda but to go back to sleep for a couple of hours.

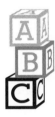

## Twin Tip

One of your twins may almost always be the baby to wake up from his nap hungry for milk. You are not scarring his twin for life by always waking him up to eat with his sibling; you are helping him by maintaining his parents' sanity. If you coordinate your twins' schedules, over time each baby's internal clock will align with the other baby's clock, and they will naturally get hungry at similar times.

Then, after a good nap (an hour or more), when one of your twins wakes up, watch the clock. If your other hasn't awoken within 10 minutes, wake him up as well and proceed with the plan again. You can see the emerging pattern. Repeating these cycles of both twins waking up, eating, burping, playing, changing, and going back to sleep is how you can handle 2 newborns at once. Manipulate this suggested schedule to fit your own needs, but make sure that you stick to your version of the schedule. Consistency is key. Babies can intuitively feel a schedule or routine, and each of you will anticipate the next step if you are consistent.

In these early days, do not expect your babies to sleep through the night. Your babies will be hungry and eager to feed frequently so that they can keep growing, especially if they were born early or weigh less than 7 pounds. While it is still too soon to expect the beautiful miracle of twins sleeping through the night, you should start taking steps from day 1 to show your babies that daytime is for playing and nighttime is for sleeping. From 8:00 pm or so, through the night until daybreak, keep feedings quiet and efficient. If possible, feed your twins in the room in which they sleep, leaving the lights as low as possible. Change their diapers only if they've had a poop or they currently have a diaper rash. Modern disposable diapers can hold a lot of urine without leaking or causing too much discomfort. After the feeding and burping, cuddle your twins a bit and coax them back to sleep. The key is to be as unobtrusive as possible. If a diaper needs to be changed, avoid too much eye contact and communication and remain expressionless. The middle of the night is not the time to play or coo with your twins. They should be getting plenty of that during the daytime hours. Although it is not for everyone, I used white noise to help my newborns sleep. A small electric fan in the room can muffle outside noises and signal to your twins that it is sleep time.

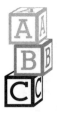

**Twin Tip**

You and your partner can be a tag team by alternating overnight feedings so that you each can sleep longer stretches at a time. For example, you can handle the midnight feeding (of pumped breast milk or formula) solo, and your partner can handle the 3:00 am feeding solo. This way, each parent can sleep 5 or more hours continuously.

## Feeding Twins: Breast Milk or Formula

Every new parent makes a decision whether to breastfeed or formula-feed her new babies. The American Academy of Pediatrics encourages breast milk as the optimal nutrition for babies up to 6 months of age, and breast-feeding is strongly encouraged for babies up to 1 year of age (and beyond, if desired). Breastfeeding has many advantages over bottle-feeding. Moms and babies have increased bonding with the physical contact. Breast milk is species-specific for your babies and is easier to digest, does not require mixing or preparation, is already at the right temperature, and contains immunologic factors that have been shown to prevent ear infections, diarrhea, and respiratory tract illnesses. For a mother, breastfeeding helps the uterus contract to its prepregnancy state. Breastfeeding moms also burn more calories to produce the milk, which can help facilitate losing weight gained during pregnancy. (Potentially delayed ovulation and menstruation are another bonus, but do not rely on breastfeeding as a sole form of birth control.) The American Academy of Pediatrics recommends that breast-fed babies receive 400 IU of daily vitamin D supplementation. Several liquid vitamin preparations for newborns and infants are available for this purpose, only requiring drops per day (always check the vitamin's newborn/infant instructions).

The decision of what to feed is not so easy, however, if you are expecting twins. You may wonder, "How on earth can I breastfeed 2 babies? Will I turn into a human feeding machine? Is it even possible to produce enough milk?" Yes, it is very possible to breastfeed 2 babies. The removal of breast milk from the milk ducts results in more milk produced for the next feeding. The demand for breast milk creates the supply. Double the demand, and you double the supply. So yes, most mothers should be able to produce enough milk for 2 babies.

If you are intimidated by the idea of breastfeeding twins, start out by learning how. See how it goes. Take it one day at a time. In the first couple of days or so after delivery, you will produce colostrum (early milk, also known as "liquid gold," that is lighter in volume but rich in immune-boosting factors). These are challenging days during which to learn to breastfeed your twins because there is not a lot of liquid for your twins to drink. The breastfeeding process becomes simpler once your milk comes in with greater volumes, usually by the fourth or fifth day after delivery (mature milk). The increased volume of milk helps your twins feel more satisfied after a breastfeeding session.

For healthy twins in the first week after birth, if your babies are still hungry after a breastfeeding session and your milk hasn't come in yet, it is OK to supplement with a bit of formula. Supplementing with 1 or 2 ounces of formula immediately after your twins have breastfed a session at each breast should not inhibit your milk production significantly. The key here, however, is that you're breastfeeding or pumping first, so as not to inhibit your own milk production. Any little bit of colostrum or breast milk your babies ingest is a bonus.

 **Twin Tale**

Despite your best efforts, because of factors outside your control, you may not be able to breastfeed. Sue, mom to third-grade twins, recalls, "I was hospitalized for a severe case of double mastitis and could not continue breastfeeding as a result. I was very worried about giving up breast milk with preterm babies; it was an unnecessarily difficult period." Be realistic and if breastfeeding is not an option for your family, know that you have other options.

If you are experiencing difficulty breastfeeding, ask for help and advice from your pediatrician, and get a referral to a lactation consultant for additional resources and support. Take the experience once day at a time, one week at a time. Try to avoid black-and-white promises to yourself or anyone else that you will exclusively breastfeed your twins for a specific amount of time, for example, up to 6 months. This is a wonderful goal, and many have done it successfully, but you'll be setting yourself up for extra stress if you try to stick to a decision that may not work. The good news is that all newborn/infant formula prepared and sold in the United States, whether brand-name or store-brand, is strictly monitored and contains all the nutritional factors that babies need in the appropriate proportions.

**Twin Support**

Any amount of breast milk your twins receive is beneficial. Do the best you can, and ask for support from your pediatrician and lactation consultant as you need it.

I was able to breastfeed my twins for 3½ months together with some formula supplementation. At that time, I made the personal choice, for many reasons, to make the switch to all formula. I will have lifelong wonderful memories of breastfeeding my twin boys on my huge twin-feeding pillow. I also enjoyed the convenience and liberation I felt when we made the switch to formula, so I've seen both sides of the story. Give breastfeeding a try. See what comes of it. If you decide to use formula, that's fine too. Again, any amount of breast milk you can give to your babies is beneficial.

## Breastfeeding Twins: How to Do It

One of the challenges of breastfeeding any number of babies is wondering how much milk the babies are actually taking in during each breastfeeding session. You will learn each of your baby's feeding patterns. One baby may breastfeed more quickly than your other, finishing up her meal within 10 minutes, while her twin lingers for more than 15 minutes. Babies who are satisfied at the end of a feeding, burp, have good wet diapers, and are passing a stool at least once a day are, in general, getting enough to eat. By the end of the first week, your babies should be having about 4 to 6 wet diapers a day and 3 to 6 stools a day. Many breastfed babies pass a stool with every feeding. This is normal and happens because breast milk is so easily digested by your babies. The best way to know whether your babies are getting enough milk is by checking their weight gain at the pediatrician's office. Especially if your babies were born small or early, you should have extra weight-check visits with your pediatrician after your babies' hospital discharge. In the early days, each baby should be gaining at least an ounce a day. At times, parents can be concerned that breastfeeding isn't going so well, but their babies' good weight gain bolsters confidence.

## Twin Support

One of your twins will likely be a more vigorous eater than your other. As long as they are both gaining weight appropriately, try to relax and avoid too many comparisons between them.

Your twins may have 2 different feeding styles, and one twin may be hungrier than your other during a growth spurt. For this reason, you may want to remember which baby breastfed on which side at each session and then switch sides for the next breastfeeding session. In alternating your twins' breastfeeding sides, you can help even out your milk supply between your left breast and your right breast so that you don't end up lopsided. In addition, your twins will benefit from lots of experience eating at both sides. Babies can at times develop a preference for just one side, and you can curb that tendency by making sure you switch sides often. You need both sides to produce milk evenly.

I had a hard time remembering who breastfed on which side when my twins were newborns, so I taped 2 note cards labeled "Andrew" and "Ryan" onto the edge of my kitchen island. I would switch the position of the cards according to who breastfed on which breast to help me remember to alternate. Even with my note card system, I would forget to alternate a few breastfeeding sessions a day, but when you are breastfeeding 8 to 12 times in 24 hours, it's OK; it all evens out. A good friend of mine wore a plastic bracelet on alternating wrists to indicate on which sides her babies should breastfeed. Smartphones have plenty of apps to help breastfeeding moms keep track of who breastfeeds on which side and when.

Take notes on your twins' feeding, urinating, and stooling patterns by keeping a simple chart. A system to document feeding information is helpful in the hospital and in the early days at home. In the chart, include the time of day, the time spent at the breast, whether you supplemented with formula afterward, and whether there was a wet or soiled diaper. Such a chart is an easy way to look at your babies' progress over a 24-hour period. You cannot rely on your memory at this sleep-deprived time in your life. Your pediatrician will want to see these notes when you visit the office in the first week after being discharged from the hospital. Alternatively, feel free to use an app on your smartphone for an electronic method of keeping track or a notebook.

If you are able to pump your breast milk, it is best to store the milk in small increments, no more than 2 or 3 ounces per bottle or freezer bag, in the early days. This method prevents waste of any breast milk if your baby is not especially hungry. If he needs more milk, you can always thaw another serving. Some moms prefer to freeze their breast milk in specially designed plastic bags. Other moms stockpile freezer-safe bottles that attach directly to the breast pump to simplify collection, storage, and feeding.

If you are exclusively breastfeeding your twins, it is important to focus on feeding at the breast as much as possible for the first 3 weeks and avoid pacifier use to prevent nipple confusion. After 3 weeks, you have a special window of opportunity, from 3 to 6 weeks of age, during which breastfed babies more easily learn to feed from a bottle without significantly interfering with feedings at the breast. Take advantage of this opportunity to get your twins accustomed to breastfeeding and bottle-feeding formula or pumped breast milk. Bottle-feeding is a great way for partners to get involved in their babies' care, promote parent-baby bonding, and give Mom a break. If you plan on returning to work after a maternity leave, you will need to train your twins to accept milk from a bottle and the breast.

How can you train your twins to feed from bottles? Provide bottles of expressed milk and the twin-feeding pillow to your partner or another caregiver. (See the next section on how to safely warm up bottles). The most important step is that you need to *physically leave the room*. Babies know when Mom is around and will prefer her familiar breast to any bottle. Be patient with your twins; it may take a few sessions for them to actually drink anything at all from the bottle.

## Formula Feeding Twins: Simplifying the Process

If you are formula feeding your babies or even just supplementing breastfeeding with formula, it is useful to make batches of formula at a time. Parents of twins simply do not have the time to prepare powdered formula at every feeding. Purchase 1-quart liquid containers and prepare 2 quarts of formula together to save time. Fill each jug with 30 ounces of formula water, and use a funnel to add 15 scoops of powdered formula (double-check with the measurements on the side of the can). If you are using concentrated liquid formula, mix equal parts concentrate and water. Warmer water may help the powder blend in more easily. Gently agitate the jug to blend in the powder. Store the jugs of prepared formula in the refrigerator, and when it's time for your twins to feed, simply pour out the desired ounces into bottles and warm them up. We found this to be the easiest way to feed 2 hungry babies powdered formula several times a day.

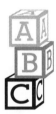

**Twin Tip**

If you are formula feeding, don't forget to use newborn slow-flow nipples to help new babies eat and digest more easily without swallowing excess air.

Microwaves are a dangerous way to warm bottles because they can create pockets of heat throughout the liquid, and the milk may be at a scalding temperature, despite feeling relatively cool when held in the hand. The safest way to warm bottles is to float the 2 lidded bottles in a large bowl of warm water in your kitchen sink for about 10 or 15 minutes before the planned feeding time. Anticipate the next feeding ahead of time and get your bottles warming so that they are ready for you when your babies need to feed.

The average number of ounces of formula needed per day depends on your babies' weights and ages. From birth to 2 months of age, each baby can take anywhere from 2 to 5 ounces per feeding. From 2 to 4 months of age, infants usually average 4 to 6 ounces per feeding; from 4 to 6 months of age, 5 to 7 ounces per feeding. After 6 months, your infants will also be eating solid foods for additional calories, so you really won't need bottles bigger than 7 ounces total. After 12 months, healthy children can transition to whole milk.

If you find a 5- or 6-ounce bottle brand and type that you like, you should stockpile the bottle. Your twins will be formula feeding every 3 hours on average, which adds up to 16 bottles a day. Decide whether you want to wash bottles frequently or in one big batch once a day. Once your twins are about 1 year of age, they will be ready to transition to drinking from a cup.

# Burping and Reflux of Twins

Whether breastfeeding or bottle-feeding, and whether prone to spit-ups or not, all babies benefit from burping breaks. About halfway through a breastfeeding session, or after 1 or 2 ounces of a formula bottle, give your twins some time to change their position a bit and burp them. Releasing any excess gas that may have gotten caught in the stomach is a good way to help your baby take the rest of the feeding. I have seen many hungry babies inhale a feeding quickly only to spit up a significant portion of the feeding because of inhaled air in the stomach. These big spit-ups often reflect *improper pacing of the feeding* or even overfeeding. Proper pacing of a feeding means giving your babies time to rest and time for any air bubbles in the stomach to rise up and be released before your babies chug the rest of the milk.

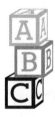

**Twin Tip**

Even if your twins are ravenously hungry, don't be tempted to feed them too quickly. You'll end up with a huge spit-up in your lap.

How long do you burp a baby after the feeding is complete? Burp your twins until they burp—and then burp them some more! It sounds silly, but so many times after the big audible burp, a smaller bubble also needs to come out. At times, you may not even hear a burp. Not hearing one is more common if you are breastfeeding, but regardless, make sure you burp each baby for at least 5 minutes. Consider the burping time to be cuddle time and enjoy it.

You *can* burp your twins simultaneously. If you are using a large twin-feeding pillow, you can seat your twins on either side so that you are hugging and burping both babies at the same time (Figure 3-4). Just make sure you've got a good hold on each of your twins, as their muscle tone is quite weak at this age. Alternatively, you can roll your twins onto their bellies and pat their backs. In this position, make sure to raise your knees so that their heads are inclined upward and the milk doesn't come rolling out of their mouths.

Twins are more likely to be born early, and babies born earlier have a greater chance of developing reflux. Reflux is what its name indicates— milk returning from the stomach, up through the esophagus (the tube that connects the mouth and stomach), and frequently out of the mouth. If your baby spits up frequently but has been gaining weight well, you needn't be too concerned. In this scenario, you may want to make sure your baby isn't getting overfed at each

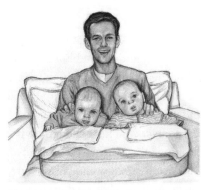

**Figure 3-4.** Burping 2 babies simultaneously using a twin-feeding pillow.

feeding and the feeding is being properly paced, with burpings midway through the feeding. If your baby spits up frequently, is fussy, and is not gaining weight (according to weight checks at your pediatrician's office), reflux may be the culprit. If you are formula feeding, your doctor may make recommendations on feeding strategies, switch your babies' formula, or prescribe a medication, depending on your baby and situation.

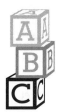

**Twin Tip**

Keep your twins upright for about 20 minutes after each feeding to help them digest their milk more comfortably.

After each feeding and burping is complete, try to not lay your baby flat immediately afterward. Imagine eating a big holiday meal and then lying flat; you would feel pretty uncomfortable. Place your twins into bouncy chairs with a 45-degree upright angle, or even wear one of your babies in a front-pack carrier if your baby's size meets the manufacturer specifications for that carrier. This way, your twins can look around and let the milk settle in their stomachs.

# Advice for Outings With Twins

For the first 3 weeks that your twins are home with you, I recommend that they lie low and stay at home. I advise this even if your twins were born full-term. All newborns' immune systems are quite immature. There are a lot of cooties out in the world! People at the mall will spy your teeny twins and won't be able to restrain themselves from reaching out to make physical contact. You have enough on your plate without your twin newborns catching a virus. Once you are out and about, be straightforward and direct with overly friendly and curious strangers. They can look, but they can't touch. A simple "Please don't touch my babies; they're getting over a cold," or a similar comment, should fend off curious strangers.

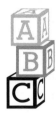

**Twin Tip**

Make sure visitors in your home wash their hands with soap and water or use hand sanitizer before holding your new babies.

Once your twins are older than 3 weeks, getting out of the house periodically is a nice way to keep your sanity. Staring at the same walls of your home, attending to the needs of 2 very high-maintenance little creatures without an occasional glimpse of the outside world, is unhealthy. A simple neighborhood walk will give everyone some fresh air. Even a trip to the drive-through post office mailbox can be a hoot if you are desperate to get out of the house. In case inspiration or necessity strikes, be ready for an outing in advance.

A stocked, ready-to-go diaper bag makes it easier to be spontaneous and take your twins out of the house. You'll have a better chance of going out if your diaper bag is ready to go. In your diaper bag, keep a plastic food storage bag with baby bottles filled with formula water, some packets of powdered formula (the kind that are premeasured—no scoop necessary), and disposable nipples. These ingredients will allow you to easily shake up a tasty meal for your twins while on the road. Of course, toss in diapers, wipes, and other necessary items.

If space permits, consider storing your twin stroller in the car trunk so that it is ready to go as well. You won't have to lug it to your car each time you need it to run an errand. It's all about simplification. If you have an older toddler, consider placing him into the twin stroller with one twin and carrying your other twin in a soft front-pack carrier. With this technique, you won't have to chase after a runaway toddler. It may be simpler to pop your twins' newborn/infant car safety seats into the stroller, if yours permits.

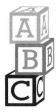

## Twin Tip

After an outing, try to restock your bag when you get a chance so that you're ready for the next trip.

In addition to your usual diaper bag, keep a special bag designated to stay in your car in case of emergency. Usually, the hospital or your pediatrician's office has plenty of freebie diaper bags that are great for this purpose. In this bag, toss a couple of bottles of formula water (refreshed periodically), premeasured packets of powdered formula, extra diapers and wipes, changes of clothes, and some receiving blankets. This bag is meant to carry extras of your babies' necessities, just in case. The emergency stash of supplies is good for peace of mind (eg, in case you ever get a flat tire while driving with your twins). It is also convenient if you're making a quick trip to run an errand and don't feel like checking the status of your usual diaper bag. You know that if your trip runs longer than you expect, you've got supplies on hand, if needed. Anything that helps you get out of the house more frequently will be good for your and your twins' sanity—a very healthy thing indeed.

# Infant Colic Times 2

What does the term *infant colic* mean, exactly? It is an older term that many people still use today to describe a newborn's or young infant's tendency to be fussy. In the past, most people believed that a lot of crying and fussiness was caused by gas pains. The current thinking is that a spectrum of *infantile fussiness* (my preferred term) may or may not be related to any gas pains. All babies are fussy at various times and to various degrees.

One of your twins may cry more than your other, depending on individual temperament. Try not to compare your babies, and don't feel guilty if you find yourself annoyed with one twin who cries more than your other. Parents of twins often feel guilty about carrying their fussier twin more often. Colicky babies have been known to endanger the very existence of one's sanity. Do your best to fairly distribute cuddles to both your babies, whether fussy or calm. You're looking to be *fair* to your 2 babies. It is impossible to give them perfectly *equal* experiences.

Newborn and infant crying tends to peak in intensity around 6 weeks and is typically vastly improved by 3 months of age. Anytime that one or both of your twins are fussy or crying, make it your routine to run down a mental list of potential triggers.

- Is your baby hungry?

- Does your baby need more burping?

- Is your baby's diaper dirty or wet?

- Is your baby cold, hot, or in pain?

- Does your baby need to be swaddled?

- Is your baby tired? Look at the clock. Has your baby been awake more than an hour and a half?

- Does your baby need to suck? Show your baby his or her hand and thumb, or use a pacifier if you prefer (after 3 weeks of age).

If your baby is still crying after you address all these issues, she is probably having a colicky moment. You may notice that late afternoon and dinnertime are particularly noisy at your house. Babies fuss more commonly during these times, in theory because the baby is worn out from all the exciting activity and stimulation during the day. Often the crying can occur a total of 3 hours a day several times a week.

Because we cannot have conversations with babies, no one knows exactly why they sometimes cry for no apparent reason. Studies have shown that the crying of colic does not seem to be related to pain. Rather, it seems to be related to a heightened sensitivity to the environment surrounding the baby. Imagine if you had been living in a cuddly, warm womb for months and were now suddenly expected to live out in the open, noisy, chaotic world. Minor sounds are like nails on a chalkboard to you, causing you to cry your heart out.

Because the crying can be related to the stimuli around your babies, the more effective soothing techniques simulate the comforting womb environment. Swaddle your twins well to mimic the tight uterine space. Walk with your babies in front-pack carriers to mimic the swaying in the womb. Rock your twins. A humming fan or even static on an AM radio can create helpful white noise. Your womb had a constant hum of activity. Imagine your babies in your uterus, with your aorta rhythmically swooshing near their heads. Although it seems counterintuitive, absolute silence can be new and upsetting to a newborn's ears.

 **Twin Tale**

**Puja, mom to boy-girl twins who are now toddlers, shares, "If the babies are crying, go through your checklist to determine the cause: hungry, sleepy, needing a diaper change, or need[ing] to be held. It's easier to diagnose the crying if you have a checklist."**

Colic seems to have one positive benefit: it can assist parent-baby bonding. Holding a crying baby close usually helps her calm down. Some have theorized that improved bonding is an evolutionary advantage of colic. Human babies, compared with most other animal species' babies, are very dependent on their parents for their care and survival. Over thousands of years, parents' ears and brains have been hardwired to respond to the sound of their babies crying, resulting in their babies surviving and growing. So even though your twins' crying may drive you crazy at times, the crying serves a purpose. It ensures that you and your twin babies will get lots of hugs every day.

 **Twin Tale**

**Lisa, mom to 9-year-old twin boys, shares, "In the first 3 to 4 months, do what it takes to get by. If [one] baby needs a binky to sleep, let him have the binky. What they need today is not what they will need tomorrow."**

We know that all babies of all cultures and ethnicities are affected by colic to varying degrees. We also know that the severity of colic has no correlation to future behavior and development. If one or both of your twins have colic, they still have just as good a chance as any other calm baby to develop into a typical grade-schooler, teenager, and adult. Don't worry that your screaming 5-week-old will stay that way forever. He will grow out of it with no harmful effects.

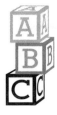

### Twin Tip

One twin is usually more "high-maintenance" than the other. Don't worry that you are neglecting your calmer twin. Relax—you may hold one twin more than your other some days, but over the months and years, it will all even out. In the long run, each of your twins will need more of you at different times.

If you are at your limit listening to the cries of your twins, you need to take a break. Enlist your partner, a relative, or a friend to watch your twins while you take a walk or a shower. Even an hour's break will help you survive this challenging period. Absolutely never shake a baby in frustration. Shaking could cause irreversible harm to your baby and her developing brain. It is OK to put a crying baby down in a safe spot (such as a crib), close the door, and give yourself a break if you are at your wit's end. Remember, your babies *will* outgrow the crying.

## Pacifier Use

Whether to use pacifiers is something that all parents must decide for themselves. Many parents happily and successfully use pacifiers and would use them again. Recent studies have shown that a pacifier can lessen the risk of sudden infant death syndrome. Remember that pacifiers need to be kept clean and available for newborns to satisfy their need for nonnutritive sucking and should be sterilized, especially if the new baby develops oral thrush, a common yeast overgrowth in the newborn period.

The upshot of a pacifier-free life is that your twins will find a way to soothe themselves. There are 2 of them and 1 of you, and you don't want them crying for you when they can't find their dropped pacifier during a night awakening. Without pacifiers, your twins will find their thumbs and comfort themselves back to sleep. Anything that helps your twins become more independent and self-reliant will help you as a parent. However, if your twins are quite fussy and nothing else seems to help, certainly go ahead and use pacifiers. Some families feel it is easier to wean babies off of pacifiers than to wean them off of a thumb, another factor to be considered in your decision.

# Seeking Support

Ask, ask, and ask for help. Try to accept everyone's offers for help. Now is not the time to be proud and try to handle everything on your own. Delegate specific tasks, such as picking up a gallon of milk at the store. Well-intentioned friends and family cannot fully understand what you're going through unless they have twins themselves. They may not be able to guess what it is that you need. If friends or loved ones happen to offer help, *take them up on it* and *be specific* in what you ask of them. Picking up diapers at the store, dropping off a dinner, or playing with your babies for 20 minutes so that you can take a shower are all specific tasks that won't be difficult for your friend and make such a positive difference for you.

 **Twin Support**

Don't underestimate the kindness of strangers. Look beyond family and friends to neighbors and your place of worship for support. Many congregations regularly organize meal delivery volunteers to help member families with newborns at home.

Depending on your level of comfort and closeness, you can also ask for assistance with overnight awakenings and feedings. Just one night of 6 hours of uninterrupted sleep will help you function much better. My dearest childhood friend visited us from out of state and offered to get up with our babies overnight so that I could sleep. I hadn't even yet taken her up on the suggestion, but already, I had felt such a wave of relief knowing that her help was available. When struggling through challenging times, it is important psychologically to know that you have help, should you need it. If finances allow, many families have found that a night nurse is a way to catch some much-needed rest for overnight twin duty. For more information, please consult the Support, Emotional, and Time-savers chapter, specifically the Seeking Support section on pages 197 to 201.

Make sure that there is a second trusted adult in your nearby geographic area who is available to help in case one twin gets sick and needs medical attention. If your partner goes out of town on a business trip, this person can be on call to stay home with your other twin and children, should you need urgent medical care for one twin. Hopefully, you will never need to use this backup, but you don't want to be caught unprepared, should something happen.

## Going to the Pediatrician

Plan in advance to have an extra pair of hands with you when you bring your twins to the pediatrician for both well-child (also known as health supervision) checkups and sick visits, whether it is your partner, a family member, or a friend. You will invariably have questions about each of your twins. Have your helper hold one baby while you speak with your doctor about your baby currently being examined. You don't want to be distracted by managing both babies at once. No one can ask important questions when one's attention is divided.

Make sure your pediatrician treats your twins as individual people and gives you an opportunity to discuss one child at length before switching gears to your other. You may have some global questions that involve both twins, but you will need time to discuss each twin independently and to have your questions about that specific twin addressed. In fact, I take care of some wonderful families in my practice who make it a priority to bring each twin separately to the office for well-child visits. I think this is fantastic!

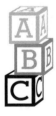

**Twin Tip**

Write your questions down on note cards or in a smartphone in advance so that you don't forget them when going to the pediatrician.

## Getting Into a Routine

After your twins' first 2 or 3 months, you'll start to see things settle into more of a routine and less of a chaotic mess. You may have 8 weeks or so of poor sleep piled up, and the exhaustion may be starting to take its toll. Your twins are going to reward you around this time with glimmers of their first social smiles.

Suddenly, all the sleep deprivation and chaos are worth it when you see these little infants smiling at you. Enjoy it and pat yourself on the back—you've earned these smiles! Now things are really going to get more fun and interesting with each passing month. Your twins are becoming increasingly aware of the world around them and are ready to interact with you and each other. Now that you have learned the fundamentals of caring for your twins, you're ready to relax a bit and enjoy the more beautiful moments of your journey with twins.

# CHAPTER 4

# Early Infancy and Getting on a Schedule

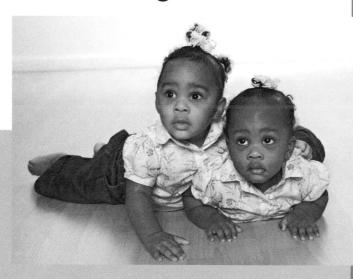

*C*ongratulations! You have survived the first couple of months with your baby twins—no small feat! Remind yourself frequently that the toughest days are likely behind you. With each passing week, you and your babies are getting to know each other more. Your babies are gaining weight each day and becoming stronger. You are learning the best ways to soothe them. They are learning to trust in you and your loving care. Your twins are comforted by the sight and smell of you, and they have grown to be aware of and anticipate your consistent love and responses on a very primary and basic level.

Your household routine is, ideally, growing more regular and consistent. A consistent home routine simplifies your life and your care of your babies. On a regular schedule, your twins know what to expect, and they are calmer in general as a result. A regular schedule benefits you as a parent as well. You know what your twins need at what times—whether it be a feeding, a burping, or a nap.

## Sleep: What Your Infant Twins (and You) Need

Around the 2-month mark, your twins may be sleeping for longer stretches at a time, but as parents, your energy levels are probably dipping. At this point, during the early infancy months, parents of twins may feel as if they are running the second half of a marathon. The end of the pregnancy was tiring enough, between a huge belly and the inability to get comfortable or a good night's rest. Now you have weeks upon weeks of sleep-deprived nights, taking their cumulative toll on your energy.

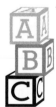

**Twin Tip**

Be proactive. Teach your babies good sleep habits now. The benefits of good sleep are well worth the effort.

Don't worry—there is a light at the end of the tunnel! Parents of twins may choose to be proactive by coaching their children to soothe themselves to sleep. A well-rested baby is a happier baby, and a well-rested parent is a more effective parent.

I'll never forget when my eldest, single-born son was 2 months of age and the sleepless nights were starting to take their toll on my husband and me—and we had only *one* baby waking up. A friend reassured us, "Oh, don't worry, my daughter started to sleep through the night when she was 9 months old." She thought she was putting our minds at ease, but the only thing I could think was, "There is *no way* I can keep living like this for 7 more months!" Thankfully, a healthy, otherwise typical baby can sleep through the night sooner than 9 months of age.

How much sleep do babies need in early infancy? On average, 2- to 3-month-olds need 15 hours of sleep in a 24-hour period. About 9 or 10 of the 15 hours of sleep should be nighttime sleep, and the remaining 5 or so hours should be divided into 3 daytime naps. Babies can start transitioning to a 2-nap-a-day schedule around the time they are 6 months of age.

The good news is that most babies can learn to sleep through the night, meaning more than 6 to 8 hours in a stretch, by the time they are 3 months of age and weigh more than 12 pounds. When a baby reaches 12 pounds, his stomach capacity is large enough that overnight feedings are no longer required. All the baby's daily calories and nutrition can and should be taken during daytime hours. With less frequent feedings at night, the baby can sleep for longer stretches. If you are breastfeeding, your body will adjust to the evolving feeding schedule.

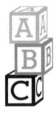

### Twin Tip

If your twins were born early or small, they will need overnight feedings a bit longer than a full-term baby would. Once your babies are more than 12 pounds, though, you can confidently proceed with sleep training.

## Sharing Space: Cribs and Bedrooms

Having a crib for each one of your twins is safer and ensures that they have the space they need to comfort themselves to sleep. Borrowed cribs that meet national safety standards fit the budget perfectly. You will be especially pleased when time flies and it is time to transition to big-kid beds. You'll be so glad that you saved the money.

Will it be more difficult to sleep train your twins if they share a bedroom? I don't think so. Your babies will become accustomed to their bedroom environment and accept the presence of their twin as part of the environment of the room. Most parents of twins have their twin babies share a bedroom because of space restraints in the home. Don't worry about the shared room interfering with your babies' learning process to sleep on their own. You do not need to buy a bigger home with more bedrooms to get your twins to sleep through the night.

It always amazes me how twins have a way of blocking out their twin's noises. Many a time, I walked into my own twin boys' bedroom while one boy was screaming his head off and my other was sleeping as peacefully as could be. It boggled my mind! Somehow, twins can shut out such overnight noises from their twin, and this skill will extend into the preschool years.

## The Science Behind Good Sleep Habits

During overnight sleep, infants and adults alike transition through various sleep stages. During these normal transitional episodes, sleep may be interrupted. Even as adults, we may not always be aware of it, but we have various points throughout the night when we are more awake than others. When we briefly awaken between sleep stages and we are in our familiar bed at our home, we can get ourselves back to sleep quite easily. However, if we are in an unfamiliar place, it can take longer to fall back asleep.

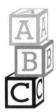

**Twin Tip**

During the process of sleep training your infants, it is important to recognize which of your twins' overnight awakenings are from *hunger* and which are a normal *awakening period* between sleep stages in which they are trying to fall asleep once again. Are your twins crying at 2:00 am? Do they weigh more than 12 pounds? If yes, don't assume your infants are hungry and automatically feed them. Give them a chance to settle themselves back to sleep.

Your twins' ability to fall asleep can be affected by a change in routine. If a parent is always present when a baby falls asleep, that baby won't be able to fall asleep without the parent. Therefore, your babies should learn from an early age how to fall asleep *without a parent present*. This also applies to babies getting used to falling asleep only in a car safety seat.

The time that your babies are falling asleep is the moment during which they need to be in a familiar setting, in conditions in which they have fallen asleep before. It is hardwired into our brains to actively help a wailing baby. If a parent always immediately rushes to comfort a baby, that baby will always require the parent's presence to fall asleep once again. If your twins are always rocked to sleep, they won't be able to fall asleep without the familiar rocking routine. If your twins typically fall asleep when breastfeeding or taking a bottle, they won't be able to put themselves to sleep without drinking milk. Give your babies lots of practice falling asleep on their own at 7:00 or 8:00 pm and they will be able to get themselves back to sleep on their own if they wake up between sleep cycles at 2:00 am.

A special note: If your twins were born small or preterm, they may still require overnight feedings at 2 and 3 months of age. But even if your twins still require the overnight feedings, use the following strategies to help them fall back asleep by themselves. As your infants gain more weight, they will be better sleepers.

## Strategies for Good Sleep Habits

Two key strategies can help your twins learn to sleep through the night.

- The first strategy is to implement a daily schedule and routine. Daytime should be filled with lots of play, interaction, and consistency in the routine.

- The second, and perhaps more important, strategy is to provide your twins with plenty of practice falling to sleep on their own. Over time, your twins will learn that daytime is for eating, playing, and interacting, and nighttime is for sleeping. When your infants are placed into their cribs *awake* at bedtime, they learn how to fall asleep on their own. Then if they wake up again at 2:00 am, they know what to do—go right back to sleep, without requiring the assistance of you or your partner.

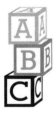

### Twin Tip

We put a 25-watt light bulb into our twins' bedroom lamp so that diaper changes would not be lit too brightly.

During the overnight hours, keep the bedroom lights as low as possible, even if your twins wake up for a feeding. Try to handle the awakening by night-light only, and turn on a soft light only if you need help changing a soiled diaper. If your infants passed stools, quietly change their diapers, but otherwise, let the diapers be, assuming your infants are not currently dealing with a diaper rash or skin irritation (for more information on diaper rash, refer to the Diaper Rash section on pages 72–73). A diaper change with all the undressing and air exposure wakes infants from their sleepy state, making it more difficult for them to settle back to sleep. Modern disposable diapers are strong enough to hold several hours of overnight urine comfortably. Keep your facial expressions as neutral as you can; now is not the time for eye contact, cooing to your twins, or rousing renditions of "The Itsy-Bitsy Spider."

When your infants realize they won't be getting much more out of you than a feeding and a burping, the only item left on the agenda is to fall back asleep.

If just one of your infants still measures underweight, go ahead and quietly and efficiently feed her as unobtrusively as you can, and then leave the room again. If you are concerned that her twin will get jealous, you can quickly feed your underweight infant in a second, darkened, quiet room before returning her to her bedroom.

### Twin Support

Good sleep habits are important for any young child and are especially critical for families with twins or more. Avail yourself of additional sleep resources if need be. *Healthy Sleep Habits, Happy Twins* by Marc Weissbluth, MD, FAAP, has advice specific for the needs of families with multiples. *Sleep: What Every Parent Needs to Know* edited by Rachel Y. Moon, MD, FAAP, from the American Academy of Pediatrics, is filled with excellent sleep advice as well. Children who are good sleepers are happy, healthy kids.

Sleep training just one infant, let alone two, is really challenging. But do not procrastinate. The longer that sleep training is delayed, the more difficult the overall process will be. As your infants grow, they will begin to develop *object permanence,* meaning that they will know you exist even when you leave the room and are not in their direct sight. If your twins are 9 months of age and aware that you are outside their closed door, sleep training will be that much more difficult. Sleep training is also more challenging if your twins are already sitting up or pulling to a stand. It is preferable to sleep train at an earlier age when your infants are more adaptable.

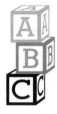

**Twin Tip**

Good sleep habits can be temporarily interrupted by an illness or travel. You will need to tend to your infants in the overnight hours if they are feverish or coughing. When everyone is healthy once again, you may need to retrain your infants to sleep through the night. If they had previously been sleeping through the night before the illness or travel, they will remember quickly.

## The Power of the Bedtime Ritual

Your twins' early infancy months are a good time to initiate a consistent evening ritual. The beauty of the ritual is that if you do it every evening, it will cue your twins that it will soon be time for sleep. If you are consistent with a bedtime routine, you will be richly rewarded in the following several years with children who easily go to bed at a healthy hour.

Of course, there will be occasions that you cannot stick to the usual nighttime routine. Sometimes you will have a date night with your partner, and your caregivers may do things a bit differently. There will be times when you'll all be out late for some fun event, and that's OK. But for the most part, do your best to keep your evening rituals as consistent as possible.

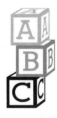

**Twin Tip**

A calm, relaxing bedtime routine sets the tone for a good overnight sleep.

An added bonus of a consistent bedtime routine is that you and your partner will have evenings to catch up with each other and to do whatever else you need to do.

When our twins were younger, the bedtime routine started with a good toothbrushing session—or, in the pre-toothed set, using a clean, wet washcloth to rub the gums. Next was a quick splash in the bathtub, and I do mean quick. Yes, we gave nightly baths, but if it is not summertime and your kid is not particularly stinky or dirty, a quick wash of the face, hands, feet, and, last, private parts will suffice. Three-month-olds are not crawling around the house picking up dust balls. You can give a quick and effective bath, all the while letting your infants explore the water, letting them learn to splash, and, in addition, cuing the approaching bedtime.

At bath time in the first 6 months, babies cannot yet sit up unsupported. We used a newborn/infant washtub and bathed our boys one at a time in succession. Save some time, water, and energy by using the same bathwater for both twins, assuming that everyone is generally healthy. After your first twin is plucked out of the tub and handed off to your partner, grab a new washcloth and get your second twin into the tub. Having supplies, soap, and towels prepped ahead of time simplifies the logistics of bath time and reduces the chances of a slip or an injury. Never leave a baby unattended in or near a bathtub. Minimize distractions and ignore the phone.

 **Twin Tale**

Brian, an adult identical twin, recalls, "My mother told us that when she gave us our first bath, afterward, she panicked because she had no way of telling us apart when we were that young. So she made her 'best guess,' and after that, she always painted nail polish on one of my brother's toes when we were infants, to help tell us apart. We then developed our individual personalities that very much distinguished us from each other!"

After the baths came pajama time and then our favorite part of the bedtime routine, story time. One parent can read to one twin while the other parent reads to the second twin. Alternatively, one parent can read to both twins at the same time. How can you read to 2 kids at once when your young infants don't have the muscle tone to really sit by themselves yet? Get creative. One way is to seat them in a comfy reading chair together and sit on the floor in front of them. Face them so that they don't fall, and hold the book up in front of them as you read. If your partner or another adult can help you, have your helper place one child onto each of your thighs in your lap, and you can snuggle and support them as you read. As you read books with your babies, they may not understand the words or images that they see in the books yet, but hearing the rhythm and sound of your voice is soothing. Over time, your twins will start to realize that the images in the books represent real-life things. It is never too early to start reading to your babies!

After reading time is finished, some extra cuddling and a little lullaby song with the lights turned off helps transition your infants to sleep. Then a fan (or white noise alternative) is turned on, your twins are laid into their cribs while still awake, and the door is closed. They may be awake for the next 30 minutes, but these 30 minutes are when they'll figure out how to put themselves to sleep.

If your infants cry after you leave the room and cannot settle themselves down, you can periodically check to reassure them and make sure they are safe. But afterward, lay them down awake in their cribs and leave the room. If they can convince you to rock them to sleep one more time, they'll always try to get you to do so. Infants should be left alone in their cribs for increasing stretches of time, with parents periodically checking on and reassuring them, until they finally learn to fall asleep on their own.

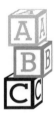

## Twin Tip

What if one parent works late some nights or all nights? You don't want your infants to miss seeing the working parent. You'll have to devise a system that works for your family. Perhaps you can compromise a couple of nights a week, giving your twins an extra-late nap before dinnertime so that they can spend some quality time with the late-working parent when that parent gets home.

Some of your friends or relatives may question your adherence to a consistent bedtime ritual. Starting good sleep habits now will extend into the next several years. Maybe your friend has only one kid and has no problem taking care of a cranky toddler at 9:30 at night who's asking for more water, but with twins, you don't have time for that situation. When you have multiples in your family, you've got to do what it takes to help them go to sleep easily. Your well-rested children will be happy and healthy and you'll maintain your sanity.

# Daytime Naps

During the daytime, remember to keep your twins' schedules coordinated with synchronized sleeping, eating, burping, playing, diaper changes, and more sleeping. Because babies can tolerate being awake during the day for only a couple of hours, keep track of the time at which your twins wake up from their nap. Of course, if both twins are not waking up at the same time, you'll need to wake up your second baby so that you can keep your 2 babies on the same schedule.

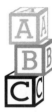

## Twin Tip

The quality and quantity of your twins' sleep is vital to your family. With good sleep habits, your twins will be happier and healthier. Good sleep boosts each baby's immune system to fend off illnesses more effectively. And if your babies sleep well, you will have extra time in your day to take care of yourself, manage necessary household tasks, and more. If you haven't quite reached this point yet, hang in there—your current efforts and strategies will pay off!

When your infants have fed, burped, played, and had tummy time, you will probably start to notice some signs of fatigue. Your infants' signs of fatigue will show you when you should scoop them up and initiate the pre-nap routine. This sends the message that sleep is coming. For the routine, you can read your infants a story, give them fresh diapers, dress them in sleepers (if you use them), and lay them into their cribs in a darkened room. At this point, they are fatigued, fed, clean, and content. What else is there to do but close one's eyes and sleep? This is the time when your twins will get practice falling asleep on their own, with their twin doing the same in the other crib across the room.

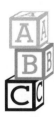

## Twin Tip

Remember that crying is a late sign of fatigue. Look for earlier clues that your twins are sleepy, such as thumb-sucking or rubbing their eyes or ears.

# Feeding Your Infant Twins

If you are still able to breastfeed your twins at this point, good for you! You may be supplementing with formula, which is perfectly fine. Any amount of breast milk your twins can get from you will be beneficial. For our family, daytime breastfeeding with a supplemental evening bottle of formula helped our twins sleep better through the night. The formula tanked them up, so to speak, and they didn't get as hungry overnight. We referred to their evening formula bottles as their milkshakes that tucked them in for the night!

If your twins are handling feedings well, experiment with a larger nipple opening. Many nipple manufacturers make a slow-flow nipple with a small hole for newborns followed by a medium-flow nipple and, finally, a fast-flow nipple with the largest opening. If you can safely use a faster nipple speed without causing excessive gas or spit-ups, you can shorten the duration of a milk feeding by 5 minutes. If you can save 5 minutes in each of the 5 feedings a day, you will have 25 extra minutes in your busy day. Simple time-saving tricks can help your life with twins get easier each month!

The American Academy of Pediatrics recommends that parents exclusively breastfeed for about 6 months, with continuation of breastfeeding for 1 year or longer as mutually desired by mother and infant. The amount of milk your babies drink at each feeding will increase as they grow. Their daily intake of milk should be about 30 ounces by 4 months of age, divided over about 5 feedings a day. Breastfed babies should continue to receive 400 IU of daily vitamin D in the form of a liquid supplement intended for newborns and infants. Mixing the batches of formula ahead of time in quart-sized jugs will continue to simplify the process of readying 2 bottles of milk for each feeding.

When your babies are developmentally ready, you can start to feed your babies solid foods, as early as 4 to 6 months of age, such as infant cereals and pureed or strained vegetables and fruits. Despite advice from older relatives, don't add infant cereal to the milk bottles to help them sleep through the night. It doesn't work and may lead to excessive weight gain. The way to help your twins sleep all night is by encouraging good sleep habits.

You will need 2 high chairs to feed your twins solid foods. High chairs have a wide range of prices. The safety seats that strap into existing kitchen chairs—the ones with an infant seat belt and eating tray—work well and are also budget friendly. In keeping with a consistent schedule for your twins, feed them solid foods at the same time and place. Place their high chairs close together, in front of you, at a 90-degree angle to each other so that they can see you and each other (Figure 4-1). Mealtimes can be a fun bonding time for all of you. Make sure to introduce only one new food at a time, waiting 3 days or so before introducing another new food, to ensure that neither infant has a reaction to the food. Store-bought baby food is just fine; pureed pears are particularly delicious. If you have time, you can also prepare food in advance by pureeing, straining, and freezing the food in ice cube trays, later popping the cubes of food out and repackaging them in resealable storage bags for safe storage. Do what works for your family.

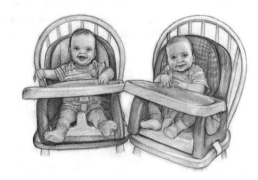

**Figure 4-1.** High chairs at a 90-degree angle to each other so that a caregiver can feed 2 infants while creating a nice 3-person social experience at the same time.

Teaching 2 infants to eat solid foods can get quite messy. In the early days, feeding solid foods once a day is a nice way to slowly introduce the concept. As your twins' skills in eating pureed foods from an offered spoon improve, you can increase the solid feedings over the next several weeks to twice a day and then to 3 times a day.

 **Twin Tale**

Do you know someone who makes only homemade baby food for her infant? Do not feel guilty if, because of realistic time constraints, your infants are eating store-bought baby food. Sue, mom to school-aged twins, states, "Work within your own boundaries of what is comfortable—and don't feel guilty about it! For me, this meant being realistic about breastfeeding, keeping extensive spreadsheets on [my] twins' sleep/feeding cycles, and ordering takeout for many meals."

Get your camera ready! Two infants learning how to eat solid foods is a real photo opportunity. Take countless digital pictures of your twins. But who is who in each picture? Other parents of older twins would tell me,

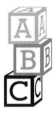

**Twin Tip**

Do not be surprised when you discover that your infant twins have different taste preferences. They are 2 unique people! If one infant is resisting a certain food, do not write off that particular food forever. Keep offering it, and over time, your infant will accept it and broaden his palate's horizon. Infants often need to be exposed to a food several times before accepting it. Ensure that you as a parent model healthy eating habits as well, even at these early ages.

"Label your printed pictures quickly because down the line, you'll forget who is who!" But somehow, in my sleep-deprived life with twin babies, I couldn't get my act together to label the pictures. What I did do, though, was dress my identical twins in theme colors. Andrew mostly wore blue, and Ryan usually wore red. My pictures never did end up getting labels, but we always know that the little guy in blue is Andrew, and the cutie in red is Ryan. One added benefit is that grandparents and friends picked up on our boys' color themes, and when they visited us, they immediately knew who each boy was without an explanation.

## Your Twins Getting Stronger

At 2 and 3 months of age, your twins are starting to develop their muscle tone. Their upper trunks and neck muscles are strengthening, and when placed onto the floor prone, they are able to start lifting their heads on their own. Parents have to become at-home physical therapists and make sure we give our twins plenty of practice strengthening their muscles.

Tummy time will help your infants gain strength and protect their heads from developing plagiocephaly, or a flattening of a part of the skull, which can partly result from frequently lying on one's back. The Safe to Sleep campaign, formerly known as the Back to Sleep campaign and introduced in 1992, has been invaluable in educating families about proper sleep positioning to minimize the risk of sudden infant death syndrome, but infants also need plenty of practice holding their bodies in other positions when they are awake and supervised by an adult caregiver.

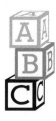

**Twin Tip**

Twins outnumber their parent; they can't be held simultaneously all day. As a result, parents of twins love the convenience of bouncy chairs or swings to entertain and contain our babies. Make sure to *avoid overuse* of such devices. Playtime on the open floor is vital and helps your twins develop their muscles and strength.

In the early stages, tummy time can be frustrating for infants and parents alike. Your infants may just cry and fuss immediately, unable to budge their heavy heads from the floor. Tummy time works best if you can give your infants something interesting to look at while on their bellies. It is an advantage to have 2 infants because your twins can face each other with baby toys between them. A mirror to look into is another popular option, but their own twin can be just as interesting! For comfort's sake, you can position a regular throw or U-shaped pillow under each twin's upper chest (Figure 4-2). It gives your twins a slightly higher and more interesting vantage point, and if one's head droops suddenly, the fall is cushioned.

*Always supervise tummy time directly.* Even if tummy time lasts only 2 minutes and you have to end it because of tears, every minute

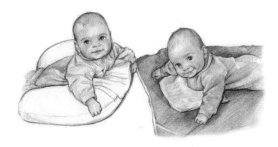

**Figure 4-2.** Tummy time fun!

counts. Try to incorporate tummy time into your daily routine of playing and eating. After a feeding and burping is a good time for tummy time. You can perform tummy time on your or your partner's chest as well, as you lean back while sitting on the couch after burping your infant. Your goal is to give your twins tummy time several times each day.

When you have twins, you can come to love bouncy chairs. The option of keeping your babies safe and comfortable while you tend to things nearby is quite a luxury. Parents of multiples, however, need to make sure that they do not overuse such containment receptacles. Babies cannot practice using their muscles if they are strapped into and confined to bouncy seats too often. You can briefly use the luxury of bouncy chairs after a feeding, for example, as the 45-degree incline can help your babies digest their milk, but after you have rinsed out the bottles and put away the jug of formula, pick your babies up and give them time on the open floor.

After the first month of age, your babies learn to visually track and follow you and other objects. They hear you coming from the next room and turn their heads to your voice. These new skills help them form relationships and interact with the world around them.

Babies usually start to roll over around 4 months of age. Rolling for the first time, however, could easily happen earlier, surprising both you and your baby. Because you never know when your twin babies will start to roll over, *never* leave them unattended in high places, such as on a bed, couch, or changing table. Consider changing your twins' wet diapers right there on the carpet floor where you are all playing already. If there is no poop in the diapers, save yourself the trip to the changing table where your attention becomes divided between your baby on the table and your baby on the floor. Injuries are more likely to happen when a parent is distracted. You will get very speedy and efficient with diaper changes!

Once your twins are 4 months of age, everything seems to get a little bit easier. Your infants get better at amusing themselves and each other for increasing amounts of time. At this age, you have time to step back, look at how far you and your twins have come, and enjoy the relative ease of these days compared with those chaotic early weeks.

## Diaper Rash

Diaper rash is common among babies after introducing solid foods into their diet. As a parent of twins, you do not have time for diaper rash! Learn how to banish it quickly so that you can move on with your lives. Be aware of the relationship between solid foods and diaper rash because some preventive care can help keep diaper rash at bay. The warm, moist environment in a diaper triggers diaper rash; unfortunately, modern diapers are excellent at retaining moisture. When changing diapers, do not rush to put the new diapers on. Give your babies' bottoms some *air time,* diaper-free, just for a couple of minutes to truly dry out the skin that is usually closed up in a diaper. One trick I used when my twins were babies was to have a few pairs of casual, comfy, all-cotton pants on hand as extras, specifically to put onto my boys when they were getting air time. The sweatpants helped catch some urine if my boys happened to pee. Warning: air exposure tends to stimulate urination!

If you have a case or two of diaper rash in your house, start using a zinc oxide cream with each diaper change. Make sure you are *generous* with the cream. Use the cream like frosting on a cake—you need more than you think. The zinc oxide creates a barrier. Many zinc oxide creams are on the market, all of which work pretty well. My personal favorite brand adds cornstarch to the zinc oxide mix, which together seems to zap the rash. If your baby's diaper rash lasts more than 2 to 3 days, or is otherwise concerning, contact your pediatrician for an evaluation.

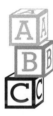

## Twin Tip

Even wipes labeled "for sensitive skin" contain preservatives that can irritate sensitive skin. Consider temporarily replacing wipes with 100% cotton balls dipped into a bowl of warm water to clean the skin during diaper rash.

Another trick I used when my boys had diaper rash was to combine air time with tummy time using waterproof pads. A strategically placed waterproof pad makes it possible to combine tummy time and air time and catch any urination that could occur without a diaper. Parents of twins learn to be quite efficient, and you, too, will learn how to multitask this way. Healing a diaper rash and encouraging upper body strength at the same time is just one example of how you can streamline your life with twins.

Certainly, if a diaper rash is not clearing up as quickly as you'd like or looks particularly worrisome, have your pediatrician check it. Some diaper rashes can progress to a yeast infection of your twin's skin, which requires a prescription medication for treatment.

# "Twinproofing"

Now that your babies are starting to move more and roll over, it is a good time to start intensively childproofing your home. Parents of twins should be extra vigilant and perform "twinproofing" of their home because twins have a way of giving each other ideas. Twins also help each other get into restricted areas that one baby alone could not have ventured into by herself. Some ideas to help you get started with twinproofing your home include

- Safety gates for the tops and bottoms of staircases

- Doorknob covers

- Electric outlet covers (that are not a choking hazard)

- Window blind cords secured out of reach

- All nursery furniture far from windows to prevent falls and from getting caught in hanging window blind cords or draperies (It is best to use cordless window products, if possible.)

- Water heater set so that water coming out of the faucet is no more than 120°F (48.9°C) to reduce the risk of scald burns

- Dressers and bookshelves secured to the wall with anti-tip devices

Always remember that even the best childproofing gadgets are no substitute for direct supervision of your twins. Do not be fooled into a false sense of security just because you have childproofed your home with all the right equipment. Dangerous things can still happen. And certain household features are difficult to twinproof, requiring parents to be watchful and vigilant. For example, a simple bedroom door can cause problems. For a time, my twin boys enjoyed a gleeful but dangerous game during which they would each push on opposite sides of the same door. A foam guard didn't work at these locations, so we had to watch our boys vigilantly and guide them appropriately.

# Returning to Work

The decisions regarding whether and when to return to work after having a child are tricky enough but even more complicated for parents of multiples. The cost of child care for 2 kids can be significant, and many families who require 2 working parents need to explore all options and get creative with scheduling.

Options for child care include an outside facility, a home-based child care provider, a sitter or nanny, or an au pair. Parents may consider working opposite hours or schedules from each other to minimize the amount of time each week that help is needed. Ensure that the outside facility or home-based child care provider maintains the proper state licensure. If you have

3 or more children, it may be most cost-effective to investigate the nanny or au pair option because your entire family will be covered, as opposed to paying an additional rate for each child. A sitter or nanny comes to a home during the required hours, but an au pair usually lives with the host family, which can be useful if one or both parents need to travel for work. Visit sites, check references, interview with prepared questions, and follow your intuition when making your selection.

Once you've determined your child care and when you'll be returning to work, make sure to make a dry run of the new routine at least a week ahead of time and make necessary adjustments. When back in a working routine, ask your caregivers to take notes on your babies' daily schedules so that you have a sense of practical matters, such as their feeding and diaper change patterns, as well as the fun stuff, such as stroller rides and book preferences. Use a routine schedule, including special rituals and time together, to share parent-child time when working parents return home. The nighttime bath or bedtime story is a perfect way for parents and babies to reconnect and bond after being apart during the daytime.

## Toys and Books

Often, the best toys for babies are the toys that do the least. If the toy does less, your child does more. You do not need to spend a lot of money on toys even though you have 2 babies who are the same age. Babies love to explore simple things such as empty, clean yogurt containers and butter tubs. Place a block inside any empty container and shake it up—watch your babies' reactions! Simple containers teach your babies about spatial relationships and help them develop their fine motor skills as they reach for a rattle placed inside a bucket.

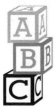

**Twin Tip**

You do not need to purchase 2 of each toy. Infant twins' typically share a developmental stage, which helps them share toys quite nicely because they won't get jealous of each other's toys.

It is never too early to read to your babies. Have plenty of board books on hand, and leave the books around the home in each room so that you can pick one up and start reading at any given moment. Your twins can also find the books on their own and eventually turn pages and leaf through the pictures by themselves. Get into the routine of visiting your local library frequently. You'll be pleasantly surprised by the board book selection for your baby twins. And best of all, the books are free. When you are feeling brave, you can bring your infants to an infant story time as well.

## Outings With Your Twins

Continue to make sure you get out of the house periodically to stay sane. Yes, there is still a world out there! Keep your diaper bag stocked so that running off on a spontaneous errand is easier. You may love your twin stroller, but consider occasionally taking your twins out with a single stroller if you have one, with a front-pack or backpack carrier. This way, you can be a little sprier on your feet by not lugging around a huge double stroller.

The single stroller-carrier combo comes in handy if you're not in the mood for everyone staring at you and your family. When people see twins, they get so excited and ask you lots of questions. Some days the attention is fun, but other days you want to just go about your business quickly. Personally, I have been told by countless strangers, "You sure have your hands full!" My standard response if I don't feel like talking? "We are very blessed," and I just keep moving along.

## Continuing to Seek Support

Do not be shy—ask family and friends for help. You are working very hard to care for your young twins, and you need breaks to stay fresh and healthy. If you do not have immediate family nearby available to help, you will need to think creatively for support. Investigate options through friends and neighbors in your community. Perhaps a family friend's preteen is interested in becoming a sitter. She can get some hands-on training by being a "family helper" within your own family. While you address other household chores, she can read to your infants. An extra pair of hands can really help you during infancy, so do not be afraid to reach out for help.

Make sure you take time to connect with your partner. A strong team works more effectively together. Communication is key, and relationships can be difficult when you're sleep-deprived. Don't expect your partner to read your mind. Ask for specific help when you need it. Stewing over an ignored household chore is not allowed. Simply talk about it in the open and ask for help in getting the chore completed.

## Twin Tale

Jon, dad to infant twins, states, "There is marital strain in any new-baby circumstance, and we certainly had our bumps upon the birth of our now 4-year-old son. But with so little downtime while tending to twins, the chances for lost patience, curt responses, and general grumpiness are big and very real—and natural—risk factors for even the greater mom-and-dad partners. I wish we'd acknowledged this prior to actually ending up in the thick of things and perhaps even had developed some strategies or 'safe words' that could more easily and quickly nip such nonproductive behavior toward one another in the bud."

# Bonding With Each Twin

Keeping your twins on the same schedule when they are young infants has many wonderful benefits; however, always keep in the forefront of your mind that your twins are unique individuals. Even at this early age, look for opportunities to connect with each of your twins. You can take one of your infants out alone for some special time, while your other twin enjoys special one-on-one time with your partner or another trusted adult caregiver. Special one-on-one time, starting in infancy, can help you and each of your twins bond and get to know each other better.

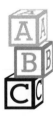

### Twin Tip

The language that you choose to refer to your twins can affect your (and others') impressions of them as individuals. Try not to refer to your children as "the twins." Instead, name them individually in conversation. Encourage family and friends to refer to your kids by name as well. If others ask you, "How are the twins?" you can respond, "Josh and Billy are great!"

When your twins are babies, you are synchronizing their schedules for survival and sanity, but always remember to regard your twins as the separate people they are. As your babies approach 6 months of age, you can somewhat start to ease out of survival mode and begin new family rituals that help you connect with each of your twins separately.

CHAPTER 5

# Later Infancy and First Birthday

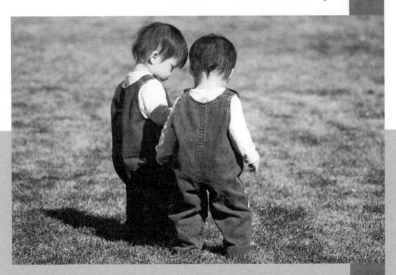

Your miraculous twins' minds and bodies grow at incredible rates from 6 months of age to their first birthday. New skills are learned at a dramatic rate. Older babies seem to learn new things *exponentially* rather than merely sequentially. Whether your twins are identical or fraternal, they continue to evolve into 2 unique, individuals. Their distinct personalities are more evident each day.

For the first time in their young lives, your babies can truly communicate their likes and dislikes to you. Sometimes, these communications may be quite crude, for example, swiping at a spoonful of food when they would rather not have another bite. Your babies will keep you guessing; one twin will gobble down dinner with an extra helping, while the other will eat a mere 1 or 2 bites and end her meal.

Your twins' smiles, coos, and early gestures form patterns of communication, which are significant to properly developing connections and relationships with others. This early communication helps your babies bond with you, your family, and each other. As you nurture your babies' growth, you will see that they are unique people, each developing at her own specific rate.

 **Twin Tale**

Jon, dad to twins, states, "In our case, the girls are fraternal, so already there [had been] an expectation of differences, but I wish I'd given more thought to these amazing individuals being thought of, and cared for, as the individuals they are versus the 'couplet' they were in utero, despite the understanding they will forever share this special bond. These days, we rarely, if ever, refer to the girls as 'the twins.' They are sisters, and yes, they are twins, but they are individuals first, each with her own traits and quirks."

## Sleep Patterns

From 6 months of age to their first birthday, babies should be sleeping, on average, about 14 hours total in a 24-hour period to stay healthy and happy. About 11 of these hours should be spent in overnight sleep, and on average, about 3 of these hours should be divided among daytime naps. The daytime sleep is usually divided into 2 naps, morning and afternoon. If you have older children, you may need to be flexible with your twins' nap schedule because of your older kids' carpooling and school activities, but do your best to be as respectful to your babies' sleep requirements as you can. If your twins get their necessary sleep, your family and daily routine will be much smoother and more harmonious.

As in early infancy, your older babies' sleep routines may be temporarily disrupted in times of an illness or travel. Once your twins are over their illness or you are back home from a trip, get everyone back on board with your usual sleep routine. Sometimes, babies can get accustomed to parents tending to them in the middle of the night if they have been congested, coughing, or feverish. When they are healthy once again, help your twin babies get themselves back to sleep. If you need a refresher on good sleep hygiene habits for your multiples, please refer to the previous chapter, specifically the Strategies for Good Sleep Habits section on pages 62 to 64.

 **Twin Tale**

As a guest speaker at a Parents of Multiples club event, I was asked how a parent could help her 11-month-old twins sleep through the night. A few weeks earlier, the mother had been concerned her daughter was getting sick and offered a bottle at 2:00 am. Unfortunately, her family fell into a pattern with this new overnight feeding, and the bottle was disrupting the daughter's and her twin brother's sleep. A healthy, normally developing 11-month-old does not require overnight feedings, and the new habit had created a learned hunger at a very inconvenient time. I informed the mother that it is appropriate to eliminate the overnight bottles. The cold turkey approach may result in a lot of tears for the first couple of nights (from both child and parent!). But with consistency, the issue can be resolved more quickly.

The strategies to encourage good sleep habits are helpful if implemented anytime during infancy, not just the early months. The difference at this stage, however, is that older babies now understand object permanence, and they know that their parents exist even when they are not in the room with them. Your babies may holler for you to pick them up in the middle of the night, or they might even resist bedtime, but I strongly recommend that you make sure you keep your bedtime and nighttime rituals consistent, assuming your babies are healthy and not currently fighting a viral upper respiratory tract infection, for example. Evening baths, pajamas, story time, and perhaps 1 or 2 songs, followed by sweet good night kisses, are what your older infant twins need to be tucked in for the night—not additional milk.

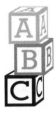

## Twin Tip

Your older twin babies are babbling and communicating more. You may notice at bedtime, after you say good night and close the door, they spend a fair amount of time "talking" with each other. These exchanges between your twins are adorable and are just one example of the special joys that parents of twins are privileged to experience. Listen at the door if you like, but don't feel the need to reenter the room and shush your babies. They are experimenting with their early language skills. They may chitchat together for a good 30 minutes or so, but as long as they fall asleep eventually, you don't need to interrupt them. For more on early language skills, please refer to the next chapter, specifically the Encouraging Language Development section on pages 125 to 127.

# Mealtime: A Whole New World

Your twin babies' nutrition from 6 months of age up to their first birthday should consist of continued breast milk or infant formula, as well as an increasing variety and amount of solid foods, beginning with purees and infant fortified cereals mixed with milk. In addition, table foods should slowly be introduced. It is hard to believe, but by the time your twins turn 1 year of age, they should be eating a diet of mostly table foods, the same table foods that the rest of your family is eating, modified to prevent choking.

If growth and development have been typical, your twins should continue drinking breast milk or infant formula up to their first birthday. Breast milk and infant formula have all the specialized nutrients in just the right proportions, which is especially important if your babies were born small or preterm. After their first birthday, your twins should be able to switch to vitamin D whole cow's milk. Cow's milk is not as nutritionally complete as breast milk or infant formula, which is why it is important that for children 12 months and older, most of the calories and nutrition should be from table foods.

You will notice that your twins' feeding patterns evolve over this period of late infancy. They may noticeably breastfeed less or drink less formula in a 24-hour period. This is typical and happens for 3 reasons.

- Your babies are eating more solid foods and are more interested in table foods. They are beginning to form taste preferences and may prefer the excitement of a new table food to the routine milk they always drink. Your twins are also mastering the art of self-feeding. Assuming they have been growing properly, as assessed at routine well-child (also known as health supervision) checkups with the pediatrician, the focus should be placed onto their increasing independence, not their total caloric intake.

- Your twins are more active and more interested in the world around them. They are working on developing their fine motor skills, perfecting their pincer grasp (thumb and forefinger closing together to pick up smaller objects), and examining microscopic pieces of fuzz. Instead of being strapped into a high chair at mealtime, they may crawl around and pull themselves up using the coffee table to see the toy sitting on top. Exploration can be a lot more fun than eating or drinking!

- All babies start to slow their rate of growth as they approach their first birthday. Because your child is not growing quite so quickly, she simply won't have the desire to eat as much as she did a couple of months earlier.

We as parents tend to worry about our kids' eating habits and wonder why a child who ate a certain amount in the past is now eating less. At this age, you need to know that drinking less milk in a 24-hour period is to be expected.

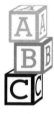

## Twin Tip

Parents of twins must always remind themselves not to compare their 2 children. Do not be surprised or overly concerned if one twin drinks more or less milk than your other. Remember that you have 2 different infants who happen to be the same age, but everyone is an individual. If you have persistent worries, check with your pediatrician. Monitoring an infant's growth on a growth chart can be immensely reassuring that all is well.

Monitor each of your babies' total intake of formula in a 24-hour period. After their first birthday, when the switch is made to whole cow's milk, you will be looking for a target maximum of 16 to 18 ounces of milk a day (definitely not more than 24 ounces in a day, which increases the risk of anemia caused by iron deficiency, as cow's milk is a poor source of iron, and if kids fill up on cow's milk, they won't have the appetite to eat other iron-containing foods). Plan ahead and make sure that you taper your babies' liquid diets if milk intake is approaching those numbers before their first birthday.

How will you transition your babies' type of milk after their first birthday? There is no one perfect answer. Some parents switch to cow's milk cold turkey after their babies' first birthday. However, some babies do not transition to a new-tasting milk so easily. For our family, I used a system of mixing formula with whole cow's milk, over time increasing the proportion of whole cow's milk to formula. I found that my kids were more willing to accept the new taste if it was introduced more gradually. Over a couple of weeks' time, change the composition of your 6-ounce bottles (eg, from 5 ounces of formula plus 1 ounce milk to 4 ounces of formula plus 2 ounces milk) until the proportion of the bottle becomes 100% whole cow's milk. This method works with minimal resistance from your twins because the taste change has been made over time. Alternatively, the cold turkey approach can work as well.

## Solid and Table (Finger) Foods

From 6 months and older, your twins should be eating new foods, meaning purees and fortified infant cereals, each week. Introduce a single new food every 3 days or so to ensure that each new food isn't causing a reaction. In the past, pediatricians recommended a specific order for new foods to be introduced—starting with infant cereals mixed with breast milk or formula, moving on to pureed and strained vegetables, and following with pureed and strained fruits, then meats, and, last, table foods. More recently, however, experts agree that a specific order of introduction is *not* required. No set order of food type is good news for busy parents of twins—one less rule that you need to stress out about! Relax, do not worry about introducing foods in a particular order, prevent choking hazards, and ensure that you are serving your twins a good variety of food groups and flavors. You are enhancing your older babies' palates, as well as providing good nutrition.

The older belief that waiting to introduce certain foods (such as peanuts) will help prevent a food allergy has been disproven by current research. New guidelines indicate that as long as you wait 3 days in between introducing new foods, you can go ahead and offer peanut, egg, and strawberry, for example, in your infants' growing repertoire of foods. Keep in mind that peanuts and all nuts are choking hazards. Even creamy peanut butter can cause choking, so offer either thinned creamy peanut butter (thinned with milk or pureed fruit) or puffed cereals that contain peanut protein. The exception to this new feeding guideline is an infant with eczema (sensitive skin, or atopic dermatitis) who requires prescription medications. Parents of these infants should consult with a pediatric allergist before introducing peanuts into the diet. The recent research is an exciting development that shows that early introduction of certain foods reduces the chance of developing food allergies.

Although the order of foods may be unimportant for your twins, a good source of iron is. Infant cereals are a great source of iron. At 6 months of age, your twins need a new, additional source of iron to accommodate their growth and red blood cell production, especially important for breastfed infants. Mix infant fortified cereals such as rice or oatmeal with pumped breast milk or infant formula (instead of plain water) to boost the caloric and nutritional value. In addition, your twins are accustomed to the flavor of the milk or formula and will happily recognize the familiar flavor in the new taste of cereal.

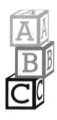

### Twin Tip

If the weather is nice, feed your babies outside as much as you can. Two babies eating solid foods can get quite messy, and life is easier if you don't have to mop up the floor after each meal. For indoor meals, some parents like to put a shower curtain or another similar tarp onto the floor underneath the 2 high chairs to streamline meal cleanup.

In addition to needing a good source of iron, your babies need fluoride supplementation starting at 6 months of age. If your home water supply is treated municipal water, your fluoride needs are most likely met. If you use well water, you should ask your pediatrician whether your twins need a fluoride-multivitamin supplement. More fluoride is not necessarily better. Babies can develop fluorosis, a condition harmful to teeth and bones, if they receive too much fluoride. Speak with your pediatrician to make sure you have the right balance of fluoride.

Your twins should be ready to try table (finger) foods around 9 months of age. To start eating table foods, they should be able to sit up fully and have a good pincer grasp. O-shaped breakfast cereal is a good first finger food because it quickly softens in the mouth, minimizing the risk of choking. To prevent choking, always cut up table foods into lengthwise, manageable sizes for your twins, and make sure foods are cooked well and on the mushy side. You may personally prefer your vegetables with a nice crunch, or your pasta al dente, but for safety during this learning process, serve your babies mushy table foods.

Do not be surprised if your twins have different taste preferences. Your babies are unique people after all. Offer an interesting variety of tastes, textures, and flavors at mealtimes. If one or both of your twins reject a food the first time it is offered, do not write off that food just yet. They may not be crazy about green beans the first couple of times they taste them, but keep trying on different occasions. Experts agree that it can take a dozen tries of a new food before a child decides that he likes it. And even from the time that your twins are babies, avoid power struggles at mealtimes.

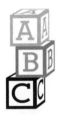

**Twin Tip**

Your twin babies love to mimic you. One day soon, they will try to feed each other!

When your babies are seated in their high chairs eating, never leave the room, even for a moment. You never know when one twin may choke on a bit of food. Sometimes, having 2 babies in the house, we can have a false sense of security, as if there is safety in numbers. Always make sure that an adult directly supervises your twins' mealtimes.

## Sippy Cup Training: Bye-bye, Bottles

Your babies will be ready to learn how to drink from a sippy cup around their first birthday. Why do pediatricians encourage families to move forward to drinking from a cup at this age? As babies grow older and become more attached to certain people and certain objects, they tend to form stronger bonds with these objects. Unfortunately, a young child may rely on a bottle for comfort in addition to nutrition, and pediatricians have seen that prolonged exposure to a bottle can cause problems such as excessive weight gain and dental cavities. If a child is sucking on a bottle habitually, the milk or juice inside can cause decay of new teeth, which is known as *early childhood caries.*

As they approach their first birthday, your children need to learn a new way of drinking milk. Milk should be enjoyed at standard mealtimes and snack times while sitting upright in a high chair or at the table. From a developmental standpoint, a child cannot learn effectively or master new skills if he always has one hand holding a bottle.

As a parent of multiples, encouraging the transition to a sippy cup is easier if done sooner rather than later. The later you make the transition from a bottle to a cup, the more difficult it will be because 1-year-olds develop their sense of autonomy more strongly each month. Changing bottles to sippy cups around the time of your twins' first birthday should help make the process more relaxed for all of you.

When you initiate your twins' sippy cup training sessions, you need to start small and work your way up. Initially, select a bottle-feeding session that is not a major feeding—maybe a midafternoon feeding. You do not want your twins to be so hungry that they get frustrated at the cup-learning process. Many sippy cup brands have a separate valve insert that is placed inside the lid to prevent spills. Make training easier for your kids and don't use the valve insert at first. These valves prevent milk from flowing freely from the spout and require that your child use more sucking action to pull the milk out (try it yourself, as you may be surprised at how much suction is needed to get the fluid moving). Not using the valve can be a bit messier, but you want to help your twins understand that this new object's purpose is to give them milk and relieve their thirst, even before they can master the proper sucking action. Trying it with an ounce of water is a great idea, because a spilled ounce of water is not a big deal. It's also a fantastic idea to get older babies (after 6 months of age) accustomed to the taste of water.

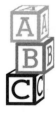

### Twin Tip

As a parent of twins, you are always on a quest for efficiency. The transition to sippy cups may initially seem like a lot of hassle or effort, and you may be tempted to keep handing your twins bottles to drink, especially if they have figured out how to hold the bottles themselves. Remember that the sooner they learn how to drink from sippy cups, the farther they are down the road to independence. When your twins are more independent, you can use your time to play and interact with them rather than to continue routine tasks of feeding and cleaning.

What about logistics? Seat your twins in their high chairs in front of you and alternate helping each child attempt to drink from the cup and playing with each child. The training sessions should be a pleasant and fun experience because you always want your children to have positive associations with mealtimes. If you find that after 5 minutes, your twins are getting frustrated or swiping at the cup, or that you yourself are getting annoyed, end the session. You can try again tomorrow. Or if one twin would rather crawl around while your other is interested and actually taking some sips of milk, go ahead and use this opportunity with your interested twin. One-on-one time with each child is always a good thing.

Several methods are available for ultimately making the switch from breastfeeding or bottle-feeding to cup drinking. Every family must choose the method that will work for them, logistically and emotionally. As with most parenting issues, no one solution can fit everybody well.

Some advise a cold turkey approach, claiming that if the breast or a bottle continues to be offered at any time of day in any way, it will cause a child to yearn and hold out for it, preventing the child from getting used to the new method of drinking. This cold turkey method is a bit harsh on parents and children. In the case of breastfeeding, it will also cause the mother a great deal of physical pain because she will likely experience some breast engorgement and leaking, if breastfeeding is terminated abruptly from 4 sessions a day to none.

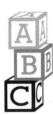

**Twin Tip**

Your twins have many transitions to make during their early years. Whether they are learning to drink from a sippy cup, toilet training, or moving to a big-kid bed, be aware of your emotions. Transitioning 2 or more kids through the same thing at the same time is tough! If you find yourself getting frustrated or annoyed, you need to take a step back and regroup. Even young babies can pick up on parental anxiety, and the transition will be that much tougher to make. Do your best to calm down, take a break, and try again another day.

A kinder and gentler approach to weaning your babies is to gradually switch the style of drinking at one session at a time until all the feeding sessions have been replaced with a cup. Start with a feeding that is usually lighter so that hunger doesn't upset your babies into being unwilling to try something new. Try this new drinking method at the same session each day for a week or so, and then select a different time of day to switch drinking styles. You can lengthen or shorten the time between additional sessions as you need, to make it work for your family. If relatives are visiting for a weekend or some other event is going on, it is fine to wait an additional week here or there to let everyone adjust to the new system. You won't want to switch a morning bottle-feeding to a cup feeding at a time when a lot of other things are happening (eg, at Thanksgiving). If you make things a bit easier on yourself, you will be a happier parent and able to help your babies get through the transition. Over time, the switch will eventually be made for all the feeding sessions of the day.

If you are still breastfeeding, you will notice that once you drop 1 or 2 sessions, your milk supply may take a precipitous dip. You may find that you will need to offer sippy cups more quickly than you had planned. Try not to fret about the total volume of milk that your twins drink. Remember that their growth rates are slowing down, and if they are truly hungry, they'll figure out a way to drink! Your twins are also eating solid foods, so they won't starve. Many breastfeeding moms hold on to one last breast-feeding session, usually at bedtime, for emotional bonding and comfort—a great ritual if you wish to continue it.

## Oral Health

Your twins' first teeth may come in, on average, around the time they are 6 months of age. Every child is different, so do not be concerned if your babies get their first teeth a little sooner or later. Ask your pediatrician about any concerns you might have. You can start using an infant toothbrush with toothpaste twice a day when the first tooth has come in. The American Dental Association and the American Academy of Pediatrics recommend that children 2 years and younger use a small smear of fluoride toothpaste, the size of a grain of rice. Just as good as a toothbrush at this young age is gently rubbing the teeth and gums with an infant washcloth and water. Get into the habit of cleaning your twins' gums and first teeth with a clean wash-cloth after feeding solid foods. Your babies are probably already quite messy with sticky cereal and pureed fruits all over their faces after a meal, and you are wiping them down anyway. Use a fresh washcloth and clean their gums and teeth first, then proceed to the rest of their faces (and bodies!). We dedicated an entire kitchen drawer to fresh, clean infant washcloths to simplify post-meal cleanups. Some families enjoy the convenience of single-use disposable wipes on their babies' faces; however, plain water and soft washcloths are a bit milder on sensitive skin and can minimize rashes.

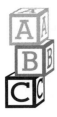

**Twin Tip**

As a parent of twin babies, you perform many of the same child care tasks each day. From time to time, step back and evaluate where you store necessary baby supplies. Could you reorganize frequently used items to make them more accessible and streamline caring for your twins?

# Play and Development

When your twins start to sit independently, usually around the 6-month mark, they will be able to view the world from an entirely new vantage point. I can promise you that your twins will achieve this milestone on different days; do not fret or compare them. My son Andrew sat up alone a full month or so before his twin brother, Ryan. At the time, I was a nervous wreck, wondering when little Ryan would sit up by himself! Now, looking back, I laugh when I remember how worried I was about Ryan's gross motor development. Today, he competes as a distance runner and swimmer in high school. Despite my concerns all those years ago, he's doing very well!

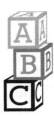

**Twin Tip**

When your twins are both sitting up independently, you can develop cool new routines that will make your life easier. For example, you can fill your big bathtub and bathe them at the same time. However, never get a false sense of security. Continue to always attend to your babies when they are in or near the bathtub and stay within arm's reach. Soon you will also be able to introduce activity centers (seats surrounded by 360 degrees of toys). Bathing both babies simultaneously or having a new fun place for your babies to spend time while you put together dinner are the sort of things that will streamline your life and make the daily routine more manageable.

A cause of concern for many parents of both singletons and multiples is wondering when their children will take their first steps. Much importance

has been placed on the walking motor milestone throughout generations. You'll often hear grandparents chuckle, "Oh, he didn't walk until
15 months," or others proudly brag, "My daughter walked at 10 months,"
as if walking made her a genius. The timing of when a child first walks
has no relation to intelligence or future motor dexterity. Walking can start
anywhere from 9 months of age to 18 months of age and still be considered
within typical range. Each child develops at his own rate, period.

Many parents' anxieties over this issue are fueled at family get-togethers
where they hear about similarly aged cousins' physical feats or at playdates
with friends because the urge to compare one's child with others is common. What is more, parents of twins have 2 cute little specimens under
their noses, and it is human nature to compare them with each other. Do
your best to avoid comparisons. Even if your twins are identical, they both
need their own time to get where they need to go. Your twin who walks
first is not better or smarter. Your one who walks later will not need special
assistance throughout her life.

 **Twin Tale**

Puja, mom to boy-girl twin toddlers, shares, "Treat your children like individuals
and don't be discouraged if they develop skills like crawling, walking, [or] talking
at different times. They will master these skills when they are ready. Our daughter
walked at 10 months, whereas our son walked at 13 months. However, our son
started babbling earlier than our daughter."

On average, twins may start walking a bit later than their similarly aged
single-born peers. I believe this is for 2 reasons. First, many twins are born
early, or preterm, putting their development onto a slightly different schedule. Second, when you have 2 children to keep an eye on, it is simply more
difficult to give them individual training sessions. Parents of just one child
have the luxury of being able to hold both their child's hands and coach him
to walk all day long, encouraging a new desire to walk with support. Parents
of multiples are not able to focus such constant attention on one child.

You don't need to feel guilty about this. Parents of more than one kid,
born at different ages, don't even have much time to devote to a single child.
My fourth child is a singleton. Did I ever have time to hold her hands for
more than 5 minutes to help her learn to walk around the house? Definitely

## Twin Support

When it comes to milestones, you may frequently find yourself comparing your twins with each other. And the comparisons won't end anytime soon. Who will count to 100 first? Who will learn to read first? Assuming your twins are generally healthy, they will probably alternate who masters a new skill first. Trust me when I tell you that in the long run, you will be amazed at how each child will take the lead in different areas and alternate being the leader. *It will all balance out.* Enjoy your child's achievement for what it is, without fretting over why her twin hasn't done it yet.

not! And she figured it out anyway. Don't worry, it will happen. But do ask your pediatrician about any special concerns you may have about your twins' motor development.

Activity centers are toys that our family enjoyed when our twin boys were older infants. These stationary toy centers have a baby seat in the center and are surrounded by colorful toys, music boxes, and activities. These can be pricey and may be too expensive for your family to buy two. We used our old one from our oldest son and borrowed one from my sister-in-law's family. Your twins can bounce safely in these toy centers, whacking the buttons on the music boxes and having fun together, and you'll know where they are—no wondering if they've crawled into the bathroom and stuck their hands into the toilet. But make sure your twins don't spend more than 15 minutes at a stretch in these toy centers. Your twins need to move about the house, developing their muscles and coordination. It was a real helper for me to have my twin boys happily and safely playing for 15 minutes during hectic times such as fixing dinner. We have hilarious home videos of our twins bouncing in tandem while giggling madly.

Do not confuse these stationary play centers with old-fashioned walkers that can wheel about the house. Walkers are extremely dangerous, and many children have broken bones or experienced serious head injuries from falling down stairs in walkers. The American Academy of Pediatrics recommends banning the sale of infant walkers. Do not buy one, and do not let any family members hand one down to you. Contrary to the old thinking, walkers do not assist a child in walking earlier. In fact, the walker uses different muscle groups than those used in natural walking and will delay independent walking.

# Language and Communication

When it comes to twins' language development, parents may hear concerning generalizations that twins sometimes have language delays compared with their singleton peers, boys more so than girls. Take these generalizations for what they are and focus on your unique children and their abilities.

How can you encourage your twins' early language skills? Narrate experiences to your twins, providing a running dialogue of the day's events, no matter how mundane they may be. "Now we're changing your diaper." "That little dog is barking."

Well before your older babies utter their first words, they have a growing *receptive* vocabulary of words, meaning they understand what you are saying even if they are not yet talking themselves. You may be mentioning a particular toy to your spouse, and your baby may surprise you by crawling over to that toy. You will notice that your twins are starting to imitate words and babble with conversational inflections, as if they are truly saying something. Encourage these early discussions, as they will evolve over time to become the real deal.

 **Twin Tale**

Puja, mom to boy-girl twin toddlers, shares, "Use baby sign language early on. It's incredibly easy to learn and will help your [babies] communicate their wants and needs before they are able to communicate verbally. Using sign language can also help avoid temper tantrum situations."

Some twins may have an early language delay because of a lack of manpower. Twins simply outnumber a parent 2 to 1, making it logistically difficult to get as much meaningful one-on-one time for talking as a single-born baby would get. The chaos in the daily household routine can make encouraging language development a real challenge. Most days, you're not so concerned with your babies' language skills as you are with trying to merely make it to bedtime with the house intact.

Unless you have 4 hands, you can change only one twin's diaper at a time. Diaper changes can be an opportunity to look into her eyes and talk to her while you change her. Her twin will get his chance when he gets his diaper changed.

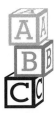

**Twin Tip**

How do you handle teaching your babies to talk while life is so crazy? Narrate the events of your daily lives. Your house is hectic—*talk* about it with your twins! "Boy, this room is messy." "Can you believe I haven't showered in 2 days?"

Studies have shown that some twins may have an early language delay, but most of these kids catch up by 4 or 5 years of age. If you have particular concerns about your twins' language development, talk with your pediatrician to determine whether further evaluation or speech therapy will be needed.

# Safety Issues

As your twins become more mobile each day, it becomes critical to make sure they are constantly supervised. Always monitor your home to make sure the childproofing is as good as it can be, and make adjustments as needed (for further information on "twinproofing," refer to the previous chapter, specifically the "Twinproofing" section on pages 73–74). There will always be areas that require protection or modification that you didn't think of, but one of your twins will helpfully demonstrate those to you! It may be a bummer to put away your wine rack for now, but good childproofing will make your life easier in the long run. A well-childproofed home allows your twins more freedom to explore and frees you from having to redirect them all day long.

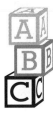

**Twin Tip**

Remember that the best childproofing in the world does not replace direct supervision. Paper clips or other small choking hazards can fall onto the ground, ready for inspection by your 10-month-olds. Your twins are little scientist-explorers, making discoveries and charting new territories, but they have little to no sense of what is safe and what is not.

Don't forget the difference between childproofing and twinproofing. Every month, your twins are getting smarter, and they will learn as much from their twin's experiences as from their own. They will each try out more things around the house than a singleton because they will try what their twin just did. Also, keep in mind that a pressure-mounted gate, which keeps a singleton baby out of a formal room full of breakable knick-knacks, may not continue to hold against the combined weight of 2 little ones leaning and pushing on it. Consider either a wall-mounted gate or a larger play yard.

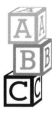

**Twin Tip**

Creatively assess your home to see whether you can create a safe designated play area for your growing twins. Safety gates come in a wide assortment and allow parents to contain babies in a particular zone. We did not have a formal living room set up in our home while our kids were young, so it was logical for us to use the space instead as a play area. Parents of singletons can get away with using a portable play yard as a temporary safe zone, but alas, parents of twins need more real estate than a small rectangle!

Now that your twins are becoming increasingly mobile as they crawl with greater speed and are learning to walk, it is nice to maintain some sort of safe zone in which to plop your twins when you cannot keep an eagle eye on them. If you have to run to the bathroom or retrieve something from the hot oven, one of your twins will find a loose button on the carpet at that exact moment and pop it into his mouth for further exploration. To prevent such an ill-timed disaster, keep a large gated play yard set up in some corner of your home.

Several options of gated play yards are commercially available; another option is to gate off a closely inspected safe corner of a room. Your twins may not spend a lot of time playing in the safe zone, but it is good to have the space prepared and ready when you need it. Keep special baby-safe toys inside, and even rotate toys into the space as needed to keep your twins interested. Inspect the space multiple times a day for surprise choking hazards that may have appeared, such as from a broken toy or an older sibling who brought his Legos nearby.

## Discipline: Working Toward Acceptable Behaviors

At this age, your twins do not need *discipline* in the traditional sense, but you do need to start teaching your twins what *is* and *is not* appropriate. It is more difficult to undo bad habits if they have been tolerated even a small number of times in the past. I have used the concept of house rules for our family. Everyone in the house must follow the house rules to stay safe. Instead of saying no repeatedly (you'll hear it said back to you often if you're not judicious with the use of the word), I try to phrase my instructions beyond a simple "No!" Instead, try, "We don't touch the oven door—it's hot." "Don't pull my hair—it hurts my head." Another strategy is to tell your children what they *should* do instead of what they *should not* do. Instead of "Stop running!" try, "Sit here on my lap."

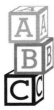

### Twin Tip

Babies' early infractions are usually just the result of early explorers acting on their natural and healthy curiosity, but parents of twins need to draw the line of what is and is not OK. The oven door window is shiny, reflective, and very interesting to an 11-month-old, but even if it is currently off, you don't want your twins thinking it is OK to lean on it and look at it up close. One of these days it *will* be hot, and you may not be right there to intervene.

When your twins engage in inappropriate behavior, intervene *immediately* so that your children connect the action with the consequence. Remove your child from the situation, and redirect your child to a new activity or location. Redirection works well because kids at this age still have a short attention span.

Do not unwittingly encourage behavior that you do not want repeated endlessly in the future. Sometimes parents are caught off guard by a pull to the hair or a bite to the shoulder by a child and, in the confusion of the moment, may have even laughed. If you laugh and say how cute it is when your twins pull on your vertical blinds when they are 10 months of age, be prepared for 2 toddlers at 22 months of age to be yanking on them regularly, unless some sort of house rule has been established early on. Your child will replicate the action to see whether she can get you to laugh again. Biting is not a great habit to encourage. Avert your face if you cannot suppress a laugh, and try to be as consistent in your responses as you can. At times, the word *no* is appropriate, if used selectively and sporadically. In the case of biting, remove your child from your shoulder and firmly say, "No. We do not bite."

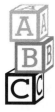

### Twin Tip

It is easier to encourage good behavior now than to have to undo bad behavior down the line.

Consistency is especially important when you have 2 kids the same age learning the house rules. Two little ones running about can quickly escalate to mayhem without parents actively supervising, intervening, and redirecting. Lessons learned at a young age will carry into the next few years and make your life easier over the long haul.

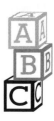

### Twin Tip

When it comes to discipline, *consistency* in your response is key. It sounds simple, but it really is not. It is much harder to be consistent when you are fatigued and overworked, running after your twins all day. There will be times when you are tired and do not feel like being on the ball, but these are the days that you still have to be on your A game and continue to enforce consistent rules.

## Your Emotions: How to Stay Sane

The constant supervision of more than one crawling, mobile baby can take a toll on parents. When your babies start crawling and walking, you will need the constant surveillance and vigilance of an air traffic controller. As with any job or task, to stay fresh, it is important to take breaks. Do not consider asking for help to be a sign of being anything less than a great parent. Consider it extremely wise to be able to identify those particularly stressful times when your whole family would benefit from one or both parents getting a break.

Ask your partner for help, who can and should be able to handle the house and all your kids for any stretch of time. Your children's father, for example, is not a babysitter—he is a parent. Do you have relatives or trusted good friends who live nearby? Is there a friendly neighborhood tween looking for "family helper" experience before full-fledged sitting? Investigate all your options for assistance.

What constitutes a break? That is up to you. You could spend an hour with a good book, take a neighborhood run, go to the coffee shop for a couple of hours, spend an evening out with friends, or take an overnight trip—it is up to you.

Asking for help and taking parenting breaks is healthy for you to step back and take a look at how your family is affecting your emotions. I have experienced a special kind of guilt starting from the time that my twins were born. When I am able to spend some time one-on-one with one boy snuggling, reading a book, or making pancakes together, there are times I cannot truly enjoy the moment because I already feel guilty that I am not spending this special time with my other guy as well. Sometimes I find myself interrupting the special moment to invite my other twin to join us, or I hurry through the moment so that I can grab that twin and replicate the moment for him. Of course, interruptions and rushing do not result in meaningful, spontaneous bonding and teaching moments. They just result in one or both twins running off elsewhere while I am left sitting there with the book asking, "Doesn't anyone want to read with Mom?" What have I learned from this? If you've got one of your twins on your lap or in your company ready for a story, *go ahead and start reading.* Over time, there will be plenty of opportunities for your other twin to get his own one-on-one time as well.

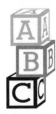

## Twin Tip

Focus on the *collection of experiences* each twin has over time. The balance will not be perfectly equal, but it should be fair. And each of your twins deserves as much alone time with you as possible. Get over the guilt and enjoy the special time. One-on-one time provides major teachable moments and encourages relationships within your family.

Especially if you are a stay-at-home parent, I'm sure that you have never felt as housebound as you have during the first year. If you were on bed rest during your pregnancy, it can add to your feelings of being disconnected from the outside world. On a certain level, it may seem easier never to leave the house again! Why would you leave? The milk is in the fridge, the stack of diapers is at the changing table, and clothes are in the drawers. Packing up your twins for any sort of outing can seem like a lot of hassle. But even if it is just a few times a month, make the effort to take your babies out of the house. It may be as mundane as walking around the mall for 20 minutes, but these experiences are healthy for you and your twins.

If you are feeling really adventurous, enlist your partner or another adult to help your family go to a local pool. It may be daunting to plan, prepare, and execute the outing—frankly, it will feel as if you are planning a small military operation—but it will be mentally energizing for all involved.

 **Twin Tale**

When our twins were babies, it was always surprising to my husband and me how calm and focused our boys were after even a simple trip to a sandwich shop. Just like for adults, taking twin 11-month-olds out of their usual environment and routine can help them refresh and refocus. They can come back to their familiar play areas and toys with a new perspective and a new appreciation.

## Finding Time With Each Twin

A child who receives plenty of positive one-on-one time will be less likely to act out in other areas to receive negative attention. Attention, whether positive or negative, is what your twins crave from you. These one-on-one moments of positive interaction are also needed so that you can start to recognize the individual and unique traits that each twin has. Even identical twins can have very different ways of looking at the world.

How can a busy family squeeze in one-on-one time with each child? Get creative and look for new ways each week. Every family needs to grocery shop periodically. You can rotate turns each week for one-on-one shopping trips with a parent. One child gets a fun outing, seeing all the excitement at the store and learning colors and numbers as you select 4 green apples to put into a bag, while your other child gets playtime with your partner at home. You won't need to feel guilty about it because the next weekend, it will be your other twin's turn to go. If a relative lives nearby, perhaps that relative can stay home with one twin while you take your other for a walk to talk about things you see in the neighborhood, squeezing in a bit of healthy exercise as well.

## Year 1: An Extraordinary Time That Flies By!

Congratulations! You have survived the first year with your twins! Take a look at your home videos and laugh at how large your pregnant belly was. Smile at your 2 beautiful children who just happened to be born on the same day, and look how far you have all come. If you are going to have a birthday party, make it a small party in the middle of the day. You won't be overwhelmed, your twins won't be overstimulated, and you can all enjoy the celebration.

 **Twin Tale**

Danielle, mom to school-aged twins, states, "Even though they share a birthday, we always had separate cakes and sang separately. As my twins get older, they still enjoy getting to pick out their own cake[s]." Take photos of each twin alone with her cake, as well as together with both cakes. You can even alternate who gets sung to first each year.

The first year flies by even faster than it does with a single-born baby because you are just so busy. Of course, you will have days when you think your twins will never sit unsupported, never hold on to a sippy cup and drink by themselves, or never talk. But then you turn around one day and everything has suddenly changed. They are now running after each other pretending to be puppies, barking loudly, and laughing hysterically.

I was too busy to keep detailed baby books, but I kept a simple book for each of them. If one of my twins did something cute, I would jot it down on a notepad. I would pile up my notes and every couple of months, I would rewrite them all at once in the books. Use your smartphone's notes function if that works better for you.

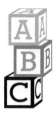

## Twin Tip

If everything is going wrong, the house is a mess, and your babies are wearing pajamas all day, every day, just laugh and enjoy it! Think of all the great stories you will have for family lore. Your children will never remember how clean your house was growing up. They will remember how much fun they had with you.

Invariably, when you take your twins out into the world, people will be interested in your crazy little family. The best encounters for me are from parents who have had twins themselves who are now grown. I remember when an older gentleman spied my husband and me eating lunch in a casual restaurant with our 2-year-old son and 12-month-old twins. He approached us when he and his wife were leaving and told us that they had twins with a closely spaced older brother and they were all grown up now. He paused, gave a sly grin, and said, "It's a lot of fun, isn't it?"

It helps to know that other people have not only survived your situation but also enjoyed it. Feeling isolated is common, especially if you are staying home with your children. Soon, the hustle and bustle of your twins' toddler and preschool years will replace the isolation you may be experiencing now.

# CHAPTER 6

# The Toddler Years (1- and 2-Year-Olds)

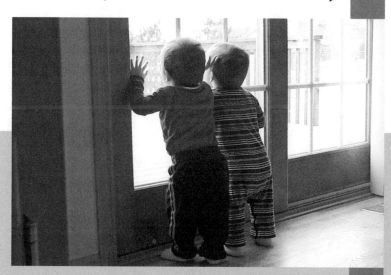

With each passing month and each passing year, life with your twins gets easier and easier. The daytime routine has an increasingly consistent rhythm and flow. Using a fairly dependable schedule, children and parents alike can predict what will happen next. Everyone will get along harmoniously with a good home schedule because everyone is on the same page. At nighttime, your toddler twins are old enough to sleep through the night consistently and regularly. The more sleep everyone gets at night, parents included, the healthier and happier everyone will be.

That said, life with twins does not become easier in a straightforward manner. The day-to-day routine gets easier, but the significant *transitions* of the toddler years provide some bumps in the road. Discipline and toilet training are 2 examples of such bumps.

Understanding the age-specific developmental milestones for toddlers as you parent children at this particular age and stage of life will help you anticipate the bumps along the way. For many toddler behaviors, parents can find reassurance in the expression "It's the age, not the child." Instead of attributing stubborn personality traits to a child with a sense of permanence, parents should remember these are developmentally appropriate stages for a child that will likely be outgrown with time, love, and nurturing. Children 1 and 2 years of age have an increasing sense of self: each child is realizing that she is a person separate from her parents and her twin. As your children have a growing sense that they are independent people, they will seek to separate themselves from their parents and twin. This independence may sometimes exhibit itself in unpleasant ways.

 **Twin Tale**

Michelle, mom to third-grade twin boys, shares, "What helped most during my sons' toddler years was keeping them on a schedule but also being flexible for changes. The routine stayed the same at bedtime: dinner, bath, and bed. During the day, I had errands, cleaning, homework with the older kids, activities, etcetera. Times, schedule, and events would change and I would get so frazzled, but then I realized, oh well. I am doing the very best I can, and I started going with the flow. I would be open with people and tell them, 'It is hard for me to get there at this time, so I might be late.' Although my intentions were there, I recognized I might not be able to commit. I had that flexibility for my own sanity. I felt as long as I was doing my best, then I needed to not worry about the other stuff."

The toddler years can be both exciting and scary for your children. Your role as a parent is to continue to provide the same loving, secure environment as you did in their infancy while showing them how to behave appropriately. Your patience, coupled with gentle encouragement, will help guide your toddler twins to mature and grow into well-behaved preschoolers. There will be some challenges during their toddler years, but try not to get too frustrated on the difficult days. Enjoy your children and watch with amazement at how quickly they learn.

## Sleep Issues

Your twins' nap time is sacred. A regular, consistent sleep schedule keeps your children happy and healthy and can save your sanity. No matter how crazy your days are, there is a predictable chunk of time each day that you know you can work on your to-do list, put away laundry, or take a nap yourself!

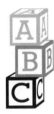

### Twin Tip

Keep in mind that every family schedule has different needs. When your twins are toddlers, you may need to shift from 2 naps a day to 1 major early afternoon nap a day because of a resistance to the morning nap or to accommodate an older child's needs. Look at your family's schedule to determine the best way to provide your twins with, on average, 14 hours of sleep each day. Parents who work outside the home may choose to give their kids an early afternoon nap until their kids are 5 years of age, so that their family can have some quality time in the evenings without their kids being overtired.

As your twins grow into toddlers with new interests and abilities, life gets more exciting and the idea of sleep becomes less appealing. Your formerly agreeable nappers may suddenly resist the idea of midday slumber. Do not mistake this disinterest as a sign that they don't need naps anymore. On average, 1- and 2-year-olds still require 14 hours of sleep every day in the form of 11 to 12 hours of overnight sleep as well as 1 or 2 naps a day totaling 2 to 3 hours in length. Every child is different, but some kids may give up naps around 2½ or 3 years of age, at which time they will benefit from quiet time (read more about quiet time in the Need for Naps [or Quiet Time] section on pages 111–112).

**Twin Tale**

Lisa, mom to 9-year-old twin boys, relates, "Be consistent with your twins' sleep. Without good sleep, you have no chance of having a good day. Be consistent with naps, bedtimes, and the routines preceding those."

If your twins are resisting nap time or bedtime, remember that overtired kids may actually have more difficulty falling asleep than well-rested kids. If your toddler twins are more resistant at nap time, you may want to consider starting nap time earlier to see whether they'll go to sleep more easily. Give yourself room to experiment to find out the best solution for your family. If your twins are particularly cranky one week, poor sleep may be the culprit. Try a few days with earlier nap times and bedtimes and see what happens. If your kids are pretty happy with the new schedule, you can be more confident that they're getting enough rest.

Some parents celebrate their children's second birthday with big-kid beds, but speaking from experience, big-kid beds will introduce a whole new set of sleep issues. Let your kids enjoy their cribs as long as possible (as long as they are remaining safely in their cribs), but be prepared for the big-kid bed transition. You never know when the day will arrive that they learn to climb out of their cribs. When one twin learns how to hop out of the crib, her twin will learn by watching her. If you don't have big-kid beds ready yet and your twins start climbing out of their cribs, a safe, temporary transition is to simply remove the cribs from the room and place the crib mattresses directly onto the floor. This reduces the risk of injuries from falls.

A reliable sleep schedule that continues as twins grow older is in everyone's best interest—the twins, parents, and siblings. When our twins were 1-year-olds, their nap time was ideal for one-on-one time with our oldest son, who was 3 years of age at the time.

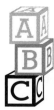 **Twin Tip**

Nap time is also a nice chunk of time to play those board games that toddlers tend to destroy or, at a minimum, mess up (the cards) and move (the players' pieces). Your twins' nap time can be the time to bring out the toys with small parts (to a designated area) that are too difficult to have around when your toddlers are awake. Everyone will become quite adept at cleaning up the choking hazards before your twins wake up from their naps.

# Transitioning to Big-Kid Beds

Transitioning our twin boys from cribs into big-kid beds was a very challenging time for our family. Even when our twin boys were still infants, I looked ahead and had a great deal of respect for, and fear of, this momentous milestone, having lived through our oldest son's transition. I recalled many nights with our little guy at our bedside at 3:00 am simply because he had the freedom to do so. I was dreading our twins' realization of "I'm free! *We're free!* No crib rails! All-night party!" Or, on the flip side, your twins might be afraid of their new environment. Switching to an open bed with no secure, tall rails can be scary for a 2-year-old. So whether your twins are elated or terrified that it's 2:00 am and they've found themselves awake in a new bed, chances are they'll do one of the following things: have a 2:00 am party in their shared bedroom, examining every nook and cranny of the room, as if they've never laid eyes on their own room before; run to you and your partner's bedside repeatedly, crying that they are scared; or a mixture of these. Such shenanigans do not lead to a good night's sleep.

In an ideal world, we would all have homes large enough to give each twin his own bedroom. However, most of us need our twins to share a bedroom for simple reasons of space. And with a shared bedroom comes all the fun of "Monkey see, monkey do."

Some families successfully try gimmicks to keep their twins sleeping peacefully all night long in their new big-kid beds. A family we know with triplets (including 2 boys who shared a bedroom) recommended that we get car beds—plastic-molded twin-size beds each in the shape of a car—for our twin boys. Apparently, their boys were so in love with their car beds that it never occurred to them to climb out of bed in the middle of the night. These car beds sounded so magical that we budgeted the steep price of 2 car beds, thinking that money toward a good night's sleep would be money well spent. To make a long story short, these car beds did not prove to be so magical for our family. We experienced nighttime parties (with draperies being pulled to the floor and night-lights being pulled from outlets, the prongs being used to "draw" on the walls), as well as the more straightforward tearful trips to Mom and Dad's bed. What works for one family may not work for another family. Because our car beds turned out not to work, we needed to implement some solid strategies to make the transition to big-kid beds smoother for everyone.

Be realistic, and remember that no matter how prepared you are and how well you are able to follow the basic principles of how to keep your kids in their own beds all night, your children are human and there *will* be some tough nights. Remember that the rough patches are just temporary road bumps, and if you follow the basic sleep rules consistently, your twins will eventually once again be sleeping peacefully each night. Illnesses, travel, and schedule changes can all affect nighttime sleep. Keep this in mind when having a particularly tiresome sleep week (pun intended). This, too, shall pass, and your kids will be on to the next milestone. In a way, the process of training your toddler twins to stay in their big-kid beds all night is like training your babies to sleep through the night.

## Strategies to Survive

There are some very useful sleep strategies to use during the big-kid bed transition. First, when your twins are around 2 years of age and are *not* quite climbing out of their cribs yet, I recommend placing a pressure-mounted gate in their bedroom doorway frame. Placing a gate at the doorway ahead of time will give your children time to get used to the gate's presence while they are still comfortable in their familiar cribs. The gate will become part of the bedroom landscape and will play an important role when the big-kid beds are in place, keeping your twins *in* their bedroom, where they should be sleeping, and preventing them from running around the house, unencumbered, wreaking havoc with no limits. The gate is especially a good idea if you are a heavy sleeper. You might not even hear your twins escape into the kitchen at 4:00 am for a free-for-all.

The next step is the selection of the new big-kid bed. Try to involve your twins in the process as much as possible. Discuss the transition often with your children. If there are older kids in your family, point out how your twins can be like their big sibling now. Let them explore their older sibling's bed. Look for children's books at your local library or bookstore about getting a big-kid bed. These steps will help your twins emotionally prepare for the change.

If your big-kid beds don't have built-in sides, you'll need to make sure your kids don't roll out of bed while sleeping. I recommend pushing each bed into a corner of the bedroom and placing a single safety gate on the exposed side. Two gates are much more affordable than 4 safety gates to protect 4 open sides.

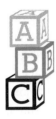

## Twin Tip

A nice idea that may work if your twins share a large bedroom is to put the big-kid beds into the room while the cribs are still there. Have both cribs and both beds in the room at the same time for a couple of days, allowing some time to talk about the change, and you can give both children a choice as to where they want to sleep at night, in the crib or in the new bed. Some kids are excited and adventurous and can't wait to try out the new bed. Other kids are a bit more hesitant and want to sleep in their familiar crib a bit longer. Both options are fine. The beauty of this method is that you are giving your twins the power to choose between 2 acceptable choices, and your children will feel empowered and more in control of the situation. At our house, our twin sons shared a small bedroom that did not have the space to use this trick. So instead, we talked about the transition frequently and let our twins check out their older brother's bed. It got to a point at which our twins were very ready and excited to use their new beds and felt in control of the situation.

Another strategy for a smooth transition to big-kid beds is to keep every other aspect of the nighttime routine the same. Bath time, pajamas, story, bed—whatever your rituals are, keep doing them. Consistent evening rituals will reassure your twins that their entire worlds are not changing, just the beds on which they sleep.

When you tuck your twins into bed, remind them that nighttime is for sleeping. "When it's dark outside, we all sleep. When it's daytime and sunny, that's when we play." Be firm and leave the room. If your twins are not falling asleep or at least being quiet, wait for 10 or 15 minutes, and if necessary, check on them to get them back into their beds. Don't give in to requests for you to lie with them unless you're prepared to spend the next 5 years sleeping on their bedroom floor. Even if you have held strong for a week, if your resolve crumples and you lie with them the eighth night, that is all your child will remember, and you'll need to start from scratch again. Use the same methods that you used when your twins were 3 months of age: check on them, be nonchalant and businesslike, tell them to sleep in their beds, and leave the room.

If they have a hard time settling down at night, you may need to start success sticker charts for sleep, one for each twin, to monitor their progress and teach them what to strive for. A night during which each child falls asleep quietly earns 1 sticker on that calendar date. After 5 stickers, for example, your child earns a small prize (your local dollar store is a perfect place to choose such a prize). Start with a low number of stickers to earn a prize so that each child has a taste of success, and then raise the bar, increasing the number of stickers to earn a prize as your twins adapt to regular sleep routines.

If, after some initial successes, your twins then start waking each other and you up in the middle of the night, be businesslike and march them back to their beds as many times as necessary.

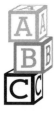

**Twin Tip**

You may be surprised to have just one child waking up a lot, while her sister sleeps peacefully through all the noise. If this happens, be grateful that only one child is awakening, and encourage her to lie quietly in her bed and fall asleep so as not to disturb her sister.

Nighttime awakenings may need to be incorporated into the success sticker charts; each twin earns a sticker for a full night's sleep. I noticed that when I used success sticker charts with my twin boys, competition set in and they became very eager to do well and earn more stickers. A little friendly competition can be a good thing if it will help everyone sleep through the night again.

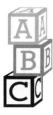

**Twin Tip**

You'll need to evaluate each twin's overall sleep pattern if rough nighttime patterns emerge. Make sure that afternoon naps do not extend past 4:00 pm so as not to interfere with nighttime sleep.

## The Need for Naps (or Quiet Time)

Later on in their toddler years, when your twins are about to turn 3 years of age and have big-kid beds, it may be a challenge for them to settle down for an early afternoon nap. Alternatively, you may notice that on the days your twins have solid daytime naps, they have difficulty falling asleep easily at bedtime. If your toddlers are approaching their third birthday and are experiencing either of these scenarios, I recommend against eliminating naps cold turkey. Instead, I recommend transitioning the early afternoon nap into an hour of enforced *quiet time,* to replace the nap time.

Quiet time is an hour during which everyone rests quietly, the TV is off and screens are put away, and perhaps one twin decides to look through a book while your other examines her right foot for a while. Quiet time can happen in your twins' bedroom, your bedroom, the family room, or whatever location works for you. You can even switch locations as need be. The important concept here is for your twins to simply relax and rest before continuing on with the rest of the day.

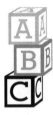

## Twin Tip

A break from a hectic schedule to rest is always a healthy idea, whether you are a child or you're an adult. If there's a younger baby in your home, coordinate quiet time with your baby's nap time. If there are older kids in the house, have your quiet time the hour before they return home from school, or encourage them to have their own quiet time to read or play with toys. An hour of peace and quiet is a precious commodity that can assist family harmony.

Each child is an individual, and one twin may still be napping well while your other is clearly finished with daytime naps. In this situation, get creative. Let your napping twin sleep alone in her room so that she is not disturbed, and take her twin into your bedroom for an hour of quiet time.

## Nutrition and Mealtimes

Feeding toddler twins can be a true adventure! You have 2 unique people on your hands. These individuals have different appetites at separate times. Each twin may have various skills when learning how to self-feed, and they may have different taste preferences as well. How do you handle accommodating your unique kids' nutritional needs in their toddler years?

After their first birthday, most typically developing children can switch from breast milk or formula to vitamin D whole cow's milk. Your twins should drink whole cow's milk from 12 months of age until they turn 2 years of age. Whole cow's milk has a higher fat content than 2% or skim, which is important for your twins' still-developing brains and spinal cords. After their second birthday, your twins can drink 2%, 1%, or skim milk.

Whole cow's milk, and all regular cow's milk, is a poor source of iron. Many kids have been known to fill up on milk and have a smaller appetite for nutrient-dense table foods, so keep track of how much milk your toddler twins are drinking each day. Your target amount of milk for each child is 16 to 18 ounces a day (not more than 20 ounces in a day, which would increase the risk of anemia caused by iron deficiency).

When feeding toddler twins, it is best to avoid power struggles. If one child is indicating that he is finished with his meal, end his meal. He may say no, shove the spoon away, or throw his sippy cup—these are all signs that you should end his meal. Do not be tempted to keep feeding with tactics such as "airplane spoons whose pilots are looking for a runway." Don't worry if his twin is still eating. Trust each of your twins' satiety centers, which tell them their tummies are full. You may have heard the expression about feeding toddlers 3 meals a day: they will "eat a meal a day, play with a meal a day, and ignore a meal a day." A key step is avoiding the temptation to offer excessive snacks or milk between meals to make up for a light meal. Toddlers who snack too much will not eat as well at regular mealtimes.

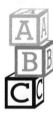

## Twin Tip

Just because one of your kids happens to be hungry that day, do not feel the need to force-feed her twin, who may not have that big of an appetite. All too often, we parents unnecessarily feel that we're not doing a good job if our kids aren't eating 3 perfect, square meals each day. However, when your kids are toddlers, you need to relax, not only for your own sanity but also to promote good eating habits. In the long run, you want to avoid recurring battles at mealtimes. Don't stress too much over a single meal. A child may not have enough vegetables, for example, but the goal is healthy eating over 2 or 3 days taken as a whole.

Appropriate portion sizes at mealtime can be surprising to parents. A proper meal is a lot smaller than one may think, especially compared with the overly abundant serving sizes at restaurants today. A serving of fruits or vegetables is 1 tablespoon per year of your child's age. A serving of protein (eg, chicken, red meat) is about the same size as your child's fist.

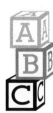

## Twin Tip

Prevent choking hazards (eg, hotdogs, raw baby carrots, nuts, and whole grapes). Make sure you slice food items lengthwise and into small pieces so that they do not block your child's airway if inhaled.

You may notice that your twins have a seemingly smaller appetite as toddlers, compared with a few months earlier. Remember that all children at this age start to slow their rate of growth. The growth rate in the first year after birth is astounding, and if your child kept that up for a few more years, he would soon be 8 feet tall!

Enjoy mealtime as a family, even when your twins are toddlers. To simplify life, families sometimes feed young twins dinner earlier in the evening, and the grown-ups eat later. And let's face it, some days can be crazy and you have to do what it takes to survive the week. However, a family meal at least twice a week shows your twins how to enjoy mealtimes and how to socially interact during the experience. Your toddler twins learn a lot by mimicking. It may seem like more work initially, but you'll see that your twins will begin to learn table manners by sitting with your family at mealtimes. Your twins will love spending this special time with you.

Serve finger foods to your toddlers, and introduce spoons and forks. Giving your twins more opportunities to self-feed is very challenging in the short run (and gets quite messy), but you'll make your family's life easier in the long run by starting utensil training early. Self-feeding is difficult for some parents to teach their kids, especially if you're a neat person. On a rushed morning, it may seem easier to simply spoon-feed the cereal to your twins. You know that they're getting the nutrition they need, and it's faster, right? But on a less-harried morning, give your kids a chance to try to scoop that cereal into their own mouths. With practice, they'll soon get there. Life will be much simpler when your twins can feed themselves an entire meal, and with practice, they will. I felt as though my twin boys would never master getting the spoonful of food into their mouths. They figured it out, *and* I found them feeding each other on a few occasions!

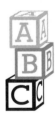

## Twin Tip

Our kids are more aware of how full their stomachs are than we are, and when we allow our kids to self-feed, they will truly eat what they need. If they're not eating much, don't sweat it. They'll make up for it at the next meal. If you have persistent worries, check with your pediatrician. A good growth pattern of height, weight, and head circumference can be reassuring.

Are you still concerned that your kids aren't eating well enough? Then ask yourself these questions. Are your twins growing appropriately, as measured at their well-child (also known as health supervision) checkups? Are they having regular, soft bowel movements, ideally once a day but at least once every 2 to 3 days? Do your kids urinate regularly? If your twins are peeing well, pooping well, and growing well, trust that they are eating well too. Relax at mealtimes, help your twins learn to feed themselves, and continue to offer a variety of healthy choices for meals and snacks.

Are you concerned that your toddler twins are picky eaters and not eating a proper *variety* of foods? Continue to offer a variety of tastes and textures each day. Model an adventurous palate by eating a healthy variety yourself. Never declare your own finicky food preferences to your kids. If you refuse to eat certain foods, of course your kids will follow suit. You can discuss the issue with your pediatrician. A daily age-appropriate multivitamin may help parents feel better about their twins' nutritional status and relax at mealtimes.

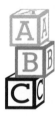

**Twin Tip**

It is pretty common for toddlers to experience occasional constipation. Switching to cow's milk and having varied eating patterns (eg, eating like a horse one day, eating like a bird the next) can have its effects on a toddler's bowel movements. Make sure your twins are not drinking too much cow's milk, which could make the constipation worse—no more than 20 ounces a day.

Offer plenty of fresh fruits and vegetables at every opportunity. If you have picky toddlers, keep experimenting until you find a fiber-rich food they love that keeps their bowels moving and their mouths happy. You can try oatmeal or steamed baby carrots, softened and sliced lengthwise, for example. Many kids adore mangoes, a very fiber-rich and nutritious fruit. Fresh apples or pears are great, and for convenience, keep canned fruits on hand such as pears, apricots, or peaches. The canned fruits tend to be nice and mushy and easy for a toddler's mouth to handle. When you find a high-fiber food that your twins love, make a mental note of it and use it as your magic bullet when you notice that constipation is starting to set in.

# Simplifying Mealtimes

Parents of toddler twins can simplify life by getting rid of their bib collection. I found that after their first birthday, messy meals never quite landed perfectly on a bib, rendering the bib somewhat useless. A spaghetti dinner with tomato sauce ends up on sleeves, in hair, and on pants. When your twins are learning how to self-feed, you can be sure food won't land on just the bib. Relax during mealtimes, and don't fret if your kids are getting messy. Keep an extra stash of clothes near the kitchen for a quick change if yogurt happens to find its way all over your kids' sleeves or dumped into their laps. When an enormous stash of bibs is given away, a drawer is now free and available to store something new.

Another mealtime change that makes life easier for parents of twins is changing infant high chairs to booster seats. Most kids around 2 years of age are ready to sit still for a meal and are balanced enough to not fall out of their chair. Every child is an individual, however, and if one or both of your twins tend to run away from the dinner table immediately, or don't have the best sense of balance, hold on to those high chairs a bit longer. Our family used wonderful toddler feeding seats that are placed onto regular dining chairs. They were slip proof, made of a comfortable foam material, did not have complicated straps, were pretty straightforward for a child to climb into and out of, and were easy to wipe clean (or stick into the sink for a deeper cleaning). An added bonus to switching to boosters: they are more streamlined and will reduce the visual clutter in your dining area.

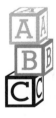

**Twin Tip**

When you're feeding toddler twins day in, day out, your children's variations in eating habits and styles may be frustrating. Remember to relax and keep your poker face on. If your kids see that they can get a rise out of you, whether it's a positive reaction or a negative reaction, they'll try again to get that reaction.

# Twins: Distinctive Individuals With a Shared Bond

Talk with any grown twins and ask about their experiences growing up and you will most commonly hear that efforts made to raise each child as an individual were appreciated. Even when multiples are at the young stage of toddlerhood, parents are wise to be aware of avoiding the tendency to parent their multiples as a group.

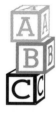

## Twin Tip

Do you have identical twins? Help extended family and friends identify who is who. Dress your twins in distinctive clothing and teach them how to introduce themselves. For example, "Hi, I'm Ryan." Your toddler twins, still quite young, probably don't realize that others can confuse them with each other. Helping each of your twins tell others who they are will minimize others' tendency to regard your twins as a unit and encourage the understanding that they are 2 separate individuals.

In the early months of raising more than one child at the same age, it certainly simplifies the daily routine to coordinate feeding and sleeping as much as possible. As your children grow into toddlers, however, each child is developing his or her unique personality and identity. Smaller steps and habits that were adopted now will grow with your children, and early efforts to treat each child as an individual now will reap rewards over the years to come.

 **Twin Tale**

Dani, who grew up as an identical twin and is now mom to twin girls in preschool, shared, "I was asked at a [Parent of Twins] club meeting (as a parent), 'Didn't you have great self-confidence since you were always with your sister?' My answer to that is if you're always with someone else, what happens when you're not with [her] anymore? Parents need to realize that just as they are raising their kids to be self-sufficient without parents, they also need to be self-sufficient without their twin."

## The Importance of Positive One-on-one Time

A child's toddler years are particularly interesting because it is the stage that she is evolving into an actual person. Sure, different infants have different temperaments and personalities, but after their first birthday, your twins are truly becoming their own person. Spending quality one-on-one time with each twin every day is important during this critical stage.

How is it possible to have daily quality time with each child if you have other children in your family? Ideally, you are spending quality time with each of your children each day, whether they are twins or singletons. There are different strategies for squeezing in quality time depending on the situation.

If it is the weekend and your partner is home, take one of your twins with you to the grocery store or on errands. Her twin can have special time with her other parent at home. Grocery shopping is something that must be accomplished each week. Multitask and combine the necessary errand with special time with your child. While you're at the store together, point out the colors of the apples you are choosing. Count out loud as you put each apple into a bag. Buying apples may seem mundane to you, but to a 21-month-old who usually has to share her parent with her twin, who rarely gets her parent all to herself, buying apples can be a real blast!

On days when both parents are home, you don't need to leave the house to arrange individual time with your kids. One parent can take one twin outside while the other parent reads with the twin's sibling. One twin can play upstairs with you, while your other twin colors downstairs with Dad. Make it a natural part of your household routine to occasionally separate your twins. Remind yourself to not think of your twins as a unit that cannot be split up.

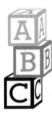

### Twin Tip

If you have to buy stamps at the post office, visit the bank, or even fill up at the gas station, bring just one of your twins with you. Ignore your cell phone and simply *be* with your child. Your child will find the trip fascinating. At this age, children do not need a theme park or a toy store to get excited.

If you are a single parent or your partner works extended hours, be sure to ask grandparents, family, and friends for assistance. See, for instance, whether Grandma can stay with one twin for an hour while you take her twin out. Think creatively and you'll find ways to squeeze in more quality time. Whether your twins are split up between you and your partner or you and a relative, each child will get a chunk of time to feel special and have an adult all to herself. Everyone wins!

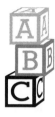

**Twin Tip**

When we create special one-on-one time with each of our twins, these are the moments that we hoped to experience when we decided to become parents in the first place. These moments are what parenthood is all about! You're not just feeding and changing diapers but *communicating* with your child in a meaningful way. With a busy house full of kids, sometimes we lose sight of that, and we need to remember to figure out what makes each kid tick. When you afford yourself the luxury of being in the company of just one of your kids, you have the pleasure of getting to know just who this little person is.

Some stressful days, to be honest, all I wanted to do was escape *alone* to the grocery store, just to think clearly and get a break from the house routine and demands. And definitely, if you feel the need to run an errand by yourself for the sake of preserving your sanity, you should. But it may surprise you to see how easy it is to take just *one* child with you to a store. Living with twins each day, you take for granted how hard you're working raising 2 or more kids. If you take just one child on an outing, you'll think to yourself, "Wow, only one kid to take care of!" The time not only benefits your child but benefits you as a parent.

How can you squeeze in one-on-one time during a busy day when you don't have the help of a second adult to care for your other twin? Look for opportunities throughout the day, and take advantage of them. Is one of your 2-year-old twins occupying himself by looking through a picture book? Drop what you're doing and quietly join your other twin to work on a puzzle together for a few moments. Let the laundry sit there—it will still be there later! Any chunk of time spent together meaningfully is beneficial for bonding and for your child's developing sense of self. If your reading twin interrupts 3 minutes into the puzzle project, it's no big deal. For balance between your twins' special time, you can steal a moment of quality time with your other twin later on.

Obviously, you'll want a balance. Make sure you're spreading the special time as evenly as possible between your twins. But remember that your twins will never have *exactly* the same amount of one-on-one time with you. It's impossible, and that's OK! You're aiming to be *fair*, but you can never make their experiences perfectly equal. If you notice that one twin has been acting out more frequently, try increasing your positive one-on-one time with him. You'll see an improvement in his behavior as a result.

 **Twin Tale**

Sue, mom to third-grade twins, advises, "Enjoy every snuggle—it goes [by] quickly!"

# Kind and Effective Discipline

Good discipline starts with good communication. When you want to communicate well with someone, whether it is your child, your partner, a friend, a coworker, or a boss, you should look the person in the eyes to convey that you are listening. Eye contact and engagement go a long way to ensure that the person you are speaking with feels validated in what he or she is trying to say. Above all, each of your twins wants you to be engaged with her.

Parents of twins have the challenge of 2 young kids at the same age, often pulling a parent in multiple different directions. Additional distractions such as smartphones, TVs, and tablets do not help matters. Even though it can be hectic with twins and siblings in your home, give your best effort each day to minimize distractions, put away the phone, turn off the TV, and truly listen to each child during pleasant interactions. Each of your twins will have a deeper connection to you, and when the time comes that your child does something she should not, your response as a parent will illustrate a clear difference between appropriate behavior and inappropriate behavior. Good communication is the backbone of effective discipline.

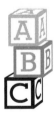 **Twin Tip**

When we discuss proper methods to discipline toddler twins, we need to define what discipline really means. Discipline does not mean the same thing as punishment. When I refer to proper discipline, I am referring to an overall household framework in which good behavior is rewarded and unacceptable behavior has appropriate consequences. Discipline takes into consideration lots of positive quality time with your child and then dictates that poor behavior eliminates any kind of attention.

## Acceptable Choices and Listening

Give your children plenty of opportunities each day to make acceptable choices. "Would you like the orange cup or the blue cup?" "Would you like the butterfly shirt or the one with the hearts on it?" Help your twins feel empowered in daily interactions by letting them select between 2 acceptable alternatives.

Above all, your toddlers want to be heard. They want to know that you love them and respect them as individuals. When your 20-month-old twins start shrieking for their sippy cups, you should calmly ask them, "What do you need? Do you want your cup? Can you ask nicely, please?" You may not feel patient enough every day to have this conversation, but if you remain calm, your children will follow suit.

If you feel your blood pressure rising with your toddler twins' demands, use some tricks to keep your cool. Imagine that you have an audience in the room with you, watching you interact with your twins, and you'll find yourself saying the right things even though you didn't think you could. Or, you can pretend that your twins are from another country and you're slowly introducing them to your language. These ideas may sound a bit silly, but it is key that you keep your cool and remain calm when disciplining your twins, even if you need to use a gimmick to do so.

Make the effort to coach your toddler twins to use their words and language instead of more barbaric behaviors. Even at this early age, if you give your child milk each time he cries for it, you are essentially teaching him to yell every time he wants milk. Start coaching him now to calm down and express himself politely. These behaviors are not magically learned at 4 years of age; it takes gentle encouragement at earlier stages from parents and caregivers.

Encourage good behavior when your twins are toddlers rather than waiting and having more issues to fix later on. In the case of toddler twins, you are coaching 2 kids how to be civilized at the same time—a lot of work, but you will reap the rewards in the long run. If you are reaching your limit (and who isn't reaching their limit when dealing with 2 sweet but at times emotional toddlers?), take a moment, catch your breath, and react as consistently as you can. You won't be the perfect parent every day, but if you can do the right thing 80% of the time, you're doing pretty well.

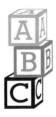

## Twin Tip

Parents of twins, listen up! Communication and relationships are a 2-way street. Just as you expect your kids to listen to and respect your house rules, you need to give your kids the courtesy of listening to and respecting them as well. To develop trust, avoid making empty promises. As an example, if you promise your child a trip to the playground after visiting the library, make sure you follow through on your promise. If you are consistent and your kids trust you, and they know you will do what you *said* you would do, your children will be calmer and more patient on the whole. It's also important to be aware of your own screen use. If you notice your toddler twins act up more frequently when you check your smartphone, consider unplugging for a bit.

If, for some reason, you are unable to follow through on promises you make to your children, address what your child says to you and acknowledge his feelings. "You're upset, aren't you? Do you wish we were going to the playground? I'm sorry we don't have time for that today; we need to go home and have lunch now." If one child is getting hysterical about something, his twin may pick up on the madness and escalate the situation. When both twins start to lose their cool, calmly call a meeting to order. Get down to your twins' eye level. Talk in a low, calm voice. Use every fiber of your being to not lose *your* cool! For instance, "We do not yell in our house. Please use your words. Dad said that it is bath time, and that means we are going to take our baths now." And most important, follow through.

## Tantrums

If one (or both, which is often the case) of your twins truly starts to melt down into a tantrum, ignore the drama and hysterics. Make sure that your child is safe and won't hurt himself or anyone else during the tantrum, and let him scream. You don't want to reward a tantrum with bribes, pleading, or any kind of attention—unless you would like to have more tantrums in your house daily, that is. Even negative attention gives toddlers secondary gain, meaning that, in that moment, they have a parent's or caregiver's full focus, and that focus can be quite attractive for a 2-year-old child. The theme of praising attention for positive behaviors, and ignoring negative behaviors, continues when it comes to navigating the inevitable tantrums.

## Consistency Is Key

Be consistent with your house rules every day, even on days when you're exhausted. Consistency is the most challenging aspect of good discipline. Sure, in theory, we all know to be consistent and have the same expectations of our kids' behavior each day, but when your twins are up all night with colds and you are about to pass out from fatigue, guess what? It's hard! Yet, you've still got to be on your A game when it comes to parenting. Whether you're having a great day or having a bad day, you still need to be consistent (as humanly possible) with your house rules so that your toddler twins learn that the rules exist, and hold firm no matter what day of the week it is.

I like using the term *house rule* with my kids because it removes the individuals from the rule. A house rule is simply the way the world works. Rules are not about what you want or what your twins want; the rules are just the way it is. When my own kids were smaller and my parents would help out, they appreciated the idea of house rules, because grandparents tend to not like to be the bad guys. They can avoid taking any blame in their grandchildren's eyes by saying, "We don't bang on the window—that's a house rule!"

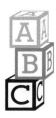

### Twin Tip

Your twins may test you when family and friends come for a visit, or when you go to a party, to see whether your reaction will be the same. Don't slack on the rules just because you are socializing. Toddlers are very smart, and if you let your guard down on a house rule just once or twice, they will remember it like an elephant and challenge you on it repeatedly. The lesson here is that the house rules are maintained even under slightly different circumstances.

## Time-outs

Once your children are around 2 years of age, they are starting to have a greater sense of what is right and what is wrong. You and your partner should discuss privately what should be considered behavior that will not be tolerated (eg, hitting or biting). All parents and caregivers need to be on the same page when it comes to proper discipline. If one of your twins hits your other, for example, declare a time-out immediately, without delay. You need to connect the offense with the punishment for your child. Your offending twin should go to a boring part of the room with no toys (we used a plain corner) or sit at the bottom of the staircase, alone, for 1 minute for each year of age. If your twin tries to escape time-out, silently march her right back. The whole idea of time-out is to remove all fun and attention.

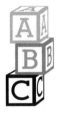

## Twin Tip

Disciplining toddlers can be very frustrating. Remind yourself that this is a difficult stage and you will get past it! Often your toddler twins may refuse to stay in their designated time-out location. If you are consistent with your rules, you will see improvement over time. Hang in there!

Avoid the urge to yell, however mad you may truly feel. Attention is attention, even if it is unpleasant and negative. Twins, as compared with single-born kids, especially crave their parent's attention, and they may actually enjoy being yelled at (on a certain level, as odd as that sounds) because they've got their parent's complete attention all to themselves. So remember, time-outs are effective only if they are used properly, meaning removing all fun and attention. When the time-out is up (an egg timer is handy to count the time), calmly get down to your child's eye level and explain why she got the time-out. Then hug and move on with the day.

If a highly desirable new toy or object is causing repeated fighting, you have 2 options. Option 1: get an egg timer and give each child a 4-minute turn with the item, and then alternate turns for each twin (adjust the timing as necessary). If the fighting is really bad, use option 2: give the toy itself a time-out. Your twins need to learn that if they can't share and play nicely with something, *no one* gets to play with it. Hide it well and try again the next day if your twins are better behaved. With consistency, your kids will learn how to play nicely, for the most part. Our kids were so used to this routine that, over the years, we had quite a few birthdays and Christmases during which presents were opened and one of our kids would immediately run for the egg timer to ensure fair turns. (You may think my idea of an egg timer is a bit dated, as many of us simply use the timer on our smartphone. I would suggest avoiding use of a smart phone, as adjusting a timer app on a phone may lead to distractions of screen time for both parent *and* child, which will undermine successful discipline.)

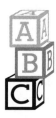

**Twin Tip**

What do you do when *both* twins have violated house rules? What do you do when both twins are hitting each other? Try not to ask, "Who started it?" If you ask who started it, it will teach your toddlers how to start blaming each other. And does it really matter who started it when they are now both hitting? They *both* need a time-out away from each other. Plan out 2 areas ahead of time. Brainstorm to see where you can create 2 safe zones for time-out sessions.

Essentially, your toddler twins are like scientists in a real-life laboratory. They perform behavioral experiments by acting differently in certain situations. They observe your reaction to their behavior and any resulting consequences, and then they register the information in their data files. If you consistently give positive attention for good behavior and remove all fun and attention for bad behavior, your twins' data files will help them make the right decisions down the line. You will have to live through a frustrating couple of years of continued research so that they can verify their findings, but if you and your partner provide a consistent framework of discipline, your scientists will emerge from toddlerhood with better manners and an ability to regulate themselves.

As a pediatrician, I warn my patients' families about self-fulfilling prophecies. If you expect a certain kind of behavior from your twins, you are likely to get it. I have often heard parents say, "Oh well, boys will be boys," letting their sons get away with more than they should. Along those same lines, there seems to be a preconceived idea of twins as being mischievous (sayings such as "double trouble" come to mind). You need to be aware of what your mind-set is. Make sure you expect the best behavior out of both of them, as if they were each single-born children. If you are inconsistent, you'll end up with twins who are hard to handle. If you have high expectations for your twins and are consistent with them, you will be rewarded.

## Encouraging Language Development

Toddlers improve their language skills by directly talking with the people in their world and by observing other people speak with each other. The most beneficial thing you can do as a parent to get your twins talking is to simply speak with each of them—a lot! Continue to narrate your lives together. Surround your children with words to help them learn how to use the words.

Many people believe in a secret twin language that only your pair of twins understands. *Idioglossia* and "cryptophasia" are both terms used to describe twin talk, or secret twin language. Personally, I feel that there isn't a secret language so much as one twin will say a word the wrong way, his twin will understand what he meant to say, and the 2 of them will continue to reuse the wrong pronunciation of the word. For example, *milk* is spoken "moak," and soon enough, both twins are calling it moak. If this happens, be supportive of your twins' attempts to talk, and repeat the correct word. "You would like miiilk? OK, I'll pour you more miiilk." Place emphasis on the correct pronunciation. Avoid saying negative things to the effect of "No, that's not how you say it," inadvertently shaming your toddlers from attempting to say new words. Just keep repeating the correct words until your twins catch on.

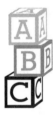

### Twin Tip

In the early talking years, some parents find mispronounced words or brand-new, made-up words to be incredibly sweet and adorable. These early words are cute. Make sure you record the invented words in each twin's respective baby book and laugh about it at night with your partner when your twins are sleeping. But in the presence of your twins, repeat the *correct, real* word back with exaggerated enunciation to help them learn. Don't perpetuate repetition of incorrect words, even if they're really funny.

On the whole, twins' language development can take a bit longer compared with that of their single-born peers, simply because they are usually sharing the same caregivers. You can't have a one-on-one conversation with each twin at the same time. Just do your best and your twins will catch up. Usually by 4 or 5 years of age, twins are talking as clearly as their peers. If you have specific concerns about one or both twins, check with your pediatrician. Don't be surprised if just one of your kids needs a language boost with some speech therapy.

**Twin Tale**

Sue, mom to school-aged twins, advises, "Take notice of any developmental delays to ensure proper treatment. My son had delayed speech due to hearing issues."

# Toilet Training

Imagine, if you dare, a new world in which you're not changing diapers all day long.... In this magical new land, you don't have to stock up on diapers every time you leave the house! Do you dare to dream?

Believe it or not, it will happen. Your twins will indeed wear under-wear one day, and they'll keep their underwear clean and dry! When will this happen? The timing of successful toilet training is ultimately up to your kids, with you and your partner's encouragement and involvement. Toileting success may not happen as early as it did for your neighbor's kid, and it may not happen by the time your kids' cousin is wearing underwear, but don't worry—it will happen. The age of a child when toilet-trained has no bearing on that child's future intelligence or status in the world. Early toilet-trained kids don't all attend Harvard. They were trained early because they had exceptional personal interest in the potty, had highly motivated and available parents who were willing and able to intensely train them, or a mix of the two.

And that's the key, isn't it? We're not talking about training just one child but two. You can do it! Toilet training doesn't happen overnight. Let's back up a bit and discuss the ages and stages that are involved.

 **Twin Tale**

Sheri, mom to twins in preschool, shares, "I wish I would have known a little more about potty training during the toddler stage. That was the hardest part of parenting by far! They're in preschool now, and things have calmed down a little."

## When and Where to Start

Start talking about the toileting process with your twins when they are around 18 months of age. Nothing intense, just the definition of terms (eg, *pee, poop, potty, flush*) and introduction of the topic. When one of your twins poops in his diaper, use it as an opportunity to talk about toilet training. If you see him straining to poop, say, "It looks like you're pooping in your diaper! Good job!" This way, he'll learn the word for what it is he is doing.

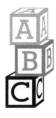

**Twin Tip**

Always be positive and upbeat about the toileting process. Toileting is a normal and natural phenomenon—*everyone poops* after all, just as Taro Gomi's well-known children's book is titled. Resist the urge to wrinkle your nose at even the stinkiest of diapers. It is important for your twins to know that pooping is healthy and normal.

Even if you are self-conscious, I recommend an open-door policy when it comes to using the bathroom in the privacy of your own home. When you need to visit the bathroom yourself, let your twins see what happens. How will they learn if they've never seen anyone else do it? Older siblings (if they don't mind) are also useful in this regard. So much can be learned by mimicking others. Anyway, when you have toddler twins in your house, you're being followed around all day as it is, so let them learn what that big mysterious toilet is there for.

You can step toilet training up a bit when your twins are around 24 months of age. Certainly, if your twins are very eager to learn, showing the signs of readiness, and perhaps trying to be more like their older sibling, you can intensify the process sooner. Just be prepared to back off a bit if one or both of your twins are showing signs of resistance. Any power struggles will only lengthen the overall process and will really test your stamina. But around 24 months, most kids are showing signs of true readiness, including walking well to a potty, positioning themselves on the potty properly without losing balance, speaking well enough to use the proper terms, and having stronger bladder and bowel control (so as to hold it to run to the potty in time). Are your twins' diapers still dry after 2 or 3 hours? That's a good sign of toilet-training readiness.

## Helpful Toilet-Training Gear

Invest in 2 potty chairs or in 1 potty chair and a ring to place onto the adult toilet seat. These could also be borrowed to save some money. Ask your family and friends whether they can give you their old ones or loan them. A good slip-proof step stool will help too. I had hoped that my twin boys would be eager to sit on a ring on the real toilet, as their big brother did, reducing cleanup work for me. Unfortunately, they were afraid to sit so high up; they preferred to be lower to the ground. So we had 2 identical potties (to prevent bickering over who got which seat) and kept them handy wherever we were spending time. In the daytime, we were mostly downstairs, so we placed the 2 potties into our main hallway (great for decorating, let me tell you), as we didn't have enough room in the bathroom for both potties. Always having a potty nearby is not so glamorous, but this is a short-lived stage, and it helps your toddlers remember them and find them easily if they get the urge to pee. We'd bring the 2 potties with us upstairs in the evening so that they were close at hand when giving baths and getting ready for bed.

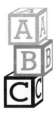

## Twin Tip

Stock up on children's books about using the potty by buying them or borrowing them from others or the local library. Reading plenty of these potty books will help ingrain the idea in your twins' heads and promote the whole idea. I refer to this as "potty brainwashing."

## Scheduling Potty Time Into Your Day

Start by scheduling potty time just once a day—a chunk of time each day when your twins sit on their potties to practice, regardless of any result. Choose a quiet time that works for your schedule so that everyone is relaxed. Make potty time fun. Read books together, sing songs, and heap on the positive attention. If you like and are able, you can give each twin her own potty time so that she gets your full attention. Your kids can initially sit on the potty chair with their clothes still on so that they get used to the idea, but soon they can take their diapers off. You're aiming for 5 or 10 minutes of pleasant practice time together. If your twins want to keep sitting longer, great, and if they run off after a couple of minutes, that's OK too. We're not looking for actual results right now. The idea of potty time is to learn that sitting on the potty is a regular part of the day and something we do every day.

Don't force the potty time or engage in a power struggle over it. If one of your twins (or both) defiantly does not want to sit on her potty chair, stop and try again another day, or alternatively, experiment with another time, such as before the afternoon nap. You'll eventually work your way up to holding potty time 2 times a day.

Is one twin clearly more interested in the potty than your other? Many parents of twins prefer to train their kids one at a time. This seems to work well particularly for boy-girl twins, as girls seem to be interested in toilet training earlier than boys, on average.

Depending on your comfort level and the degree of success you're seeing at potty time, you can make a big production of selecting some big-kid underwear at the store. Subsequently, you can start having underwear time each day, starting with a couple of hours' worth and increasing from there. In our house, we had our underwear time every afternoon starting after the afternoon nap and lasting to bath time before bed. Every hour of underwear time, check in with each twin to ask if she needs to use the potty, "to keep your underwear clean and dry."

## Motivational Tools

Success sticker charts, or potty charts, work really well for toilet training and help kids feel special. You can buy 2 big, blank poster boards at the store. Have each twin choose a distinct color, and hang the posters in a central location of your home where everyone can see them clearly.

Make a big production of writing each twin's name at the top of each poster, and draw a row of small squares at the top. Start small and make this first row only 3 squares long. Each square will get filled with a sticker (1 sticker for peeing on the potty, 2 stickers for pooping on the potty—small reward sticker collections are easily found online or at discount stores), and when the row of squares is filled with stickers, your child can choose a small prize. The first row should be short so that your child can have an early taste of success, and the following rows can have progressively more squares to raise the bar.

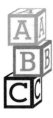

### Twin Tip

Our sons' potty charts were taped to the side of our kitchen island. Displayed potty charts are not going to be the next great idea in the world of kitchen design, but toilet training is a temporary situation, and our boys could watch their progress unfold at eye level in a central location in our home, encouraging them toward more success.

Some families use candy rewards during the toilet-training process; however, I warn against this. Food rewards, even if given with good intentions, can unfortunately send an unhealthy message to your kids by fostering an attitude about treats that can contribute to weight problems in the future. The potty charts may require a bit more effort than just handing out candy, but the beauty of the potty charts is that your kids can visualize all their success and see how far they've come. The charts can be a real confidence builder. See what works for your family.

Toileting accidents (wetting or soiling) will happen. Expect them and be prepared for them so that you are not caught off guard. Keep extra-absorbent cloths handy to help clean up pee or poop. Burp cloths from infancy are great for this purpose. Have extra wet wipes handy. When accidents happen, do your best to keep your cool. Remain calm and have your child help you clean up the pee or poop in an age-appropriate way by giving her an extra cloth to wipe the floor. Teach your twins to put their dirty pants into a bin in the laundry area *themselves* and where to get clean pants *themselves.* You want each child to understand how much easier and simpler it is to simply pee and poop into the potty. We kept a shelf nearby stocked with burp cloths, extra underwear, and extra pants just to make cleaning up after the inevitable accidents easier to handle.

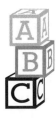

**Twin Tip**

Expect setbacks, and don't be discouraged by them. Illnesses, changes in the daily schedule, travel, a new baby—all can cause a temporary regression in toilet training. If your toddler twins have issues withholding painful poops and progressive constipation, consult with your pediatrician. Continue to be upbeat and positive, and your twins will recover. When you're worried, just remember, they won't be attending high school in diapers. I promise!

Toilet training is truly complete when each child makes it to the potty in time with *no* reminders from a parent or caregiver. When you're seeing that your kids are doing well, try to back off on the reminders, so that they can learn to remind themselves.

There are plumbing secrets every parent of twins should know. Toilet training twins is quite a task, and parents should take any help they can get. When I was training my identical twin boys, I purchased some wipes from the store. The box was clearly labeled "flushable" wipes. Anything that simplified the process of helping 2 little ones learn the language of the toilet seemed like a good idea to me.

Not coincidentally, 2 months into the toilet-training process, some unwelcome events occurred in our home. During the washing machine's spin cycle, water began gurgling in a shower drain. Long story short: those flushable wipes had collected and clogged up the main sewer line exiting the house.

As the plumber worked on the expensive repairs, he recommended not flushing anything other than poop and toilet paper—not even facial tissue. When I asked specifically about flushable wipes, he said there is no such thing, even if the box is labeled as such. If used, they should be thrown into the trash. A friend experienced a similar situation. Her plumber joked that flushable wipes kept him in business! We compared notes and figured it was time to spread the word to others with young children, especially those who are toilet training twins. Here's hoping this story keeps your pipes clear and spares you unnecessary plumbing repairs.

## Safety Issues

Continually reevaluate the childproofing in your home. Watch out for choking hazards that may have found their way into your twins' play areas. Your twins may be older now, but they may still decide to explore a small, unknown item by putting it into their mouths.

As your twins grow bigger, their style of play changes. They are faster and stronger than when they were 13-month-olds. Two or more children chasing each other can get hurt more than just one child playing alone. Are there hazards in your home that you didn't even realize were a problem? If a part of your home comes to your attention as unsafe, correct it before someone gets injured. When our twin boys were toddlers, they both fell on separate occasions, hitting the very same wall corner in a high-traffic hallway. Ryan tripped into it, turning his forehead into one big bruised egg, and several months later, Andrew ran into it playing in an exciting game of hide-and-seek, splitting his upper lip. The day after Andrew received his stitches, I purchased long foam cushions, which were made to childproof coffee tables, and taped them onto the wall corners in our high-traffic hallway. The padded-corner look may not appear in home-decorating magazines anytime soon, but we rested a little easier knowing that lightning wouldn't strike at that spot a third time.

Now that your twins are walking toddlers, you'll be spending more time outdoors. Teach your twins basic outdoor rules, such as staying with a parent and not running into the street. A fenced-in yard is wonderful for containing your active toddler twins. If a fence is not an option, monitor your twins' locations diligently. Don't get a false sense of security when other adults are present. Always make sure that both toddlers are being monitored when spending time outside.

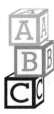

**Twin Tip**

Playing outside in the yard can be very stressful for parents of toddler twins. The minute you go outside, one runs in one direction and your other runs in the opposite direction. Brainstorm different ways to enjoy the outdoors safely with your twins. I wanted the option to have family meals outdoors. Our solution was to install child safety gates to block off the deck openings to the beckoning yard. The gates weren't aesthetically pleasing, but they were worth it to enjoy family dinners outside without worrying about 2 toddlers trying to escape. We ended up eating outdoors quite often!

Both toddlers in the kitchen brings up safety issues. As with all ages and stages, no magical childproofing gadget or gizmo can replace direct supervision. Parents need to keep a vigilant watch over toddlers when cooking. Parents can teach kitchen safety skills in an age-appropriate way. I usually kept my instructions clear and simple and defined certain tasks as "a grown-up job" (eg, slicing onions, peeling pears) or "a kid job" (eg, measuring or adding sugar, sprinkling cheese). As your children grow and develop, they'll be able to add to their repertoire of cooking tasks. From the outset, establish clear boundaries with hot stoves, sharp knives, and other dangerous aspects of the kitchen. Over time, with consistent parental guidance, your kids will learn the basics of staying safe while cooking and you'll be able to shift more attention toward the dish at hand. Some lessons will be unexpected but memorable nonetheless. A couple years ago, I gave myself a minor cut (requiring only a bandage) when slicing vegetables. One of my twins witnessed the event, and for the next couple years, if I happened to pick up any tool that had a remotely sharp edge to it (eg, scissors, knives, even a stapler), he would remind me, "Be careful with that, Mom!" In addition to kitchen safety, teach good hygiene by reminding your kids to wash their hands with soap and water before handling food and to sneeze into their "cough pocket" (crook of their elbow), not into the salad bowl.

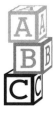

## Twin Tip

When you whip up a quick meal or tasty snack, are you bombarded by your 2-year-old twins begging, "I help you?" A while back, I posted an item on my blog about kitchen safety and was asked by a reader whether I had more tricks to share about incorporating a crowd of little kids into the kitchen. My advice? Take advantage of your kids' helpful instincts! By simply cooking together, your children can learn healthy eating habits, life skills, family traditions, and much more all at the same time—a true high yield activity. Looking at recipes and measuring ingredients boosts early reading and math skills in a very fun, hands-on way with edible results. Do you have picky eaters? Kids who play a role in the cooking process are more likely to try new foods.

What is the safest way to help your toddlers or preschoolers work at a standard counter height? Typical step stools are usually not high enough, but pushing dining room chairs into the cooking area can be both cumbersome and dangerous. Wiggly little feet in socks standing on a chair can easily slip and fall. Since our twins have older and younger siblings very close in age, we invested in a sturdy and stable step stool made specifically for 2 children to use at once. It had a rail around all 4 sides, was nearly impossible to tip over, allowed step height to be adjusted as our kids grew, and could even double as a puppet theater, if curtains were added. I used to store ours in a closet, lugging it out each day, and then realized life would be easier if we simply kept it out and available in the corner of the kitchen. It was a bit of an eyesore, but we've consciously prioritized our children's development over aesthetic appearances. (Search for "the learning tower" on the internet to see some examples. Many vendors now carry it at different price points, so shop carefully if you choose to make this investment.) When you have twins, it is worth the cost of a couple meals out in a restaurant (and is healthier) to have the ability to safely cook with your children at home over the years.

# Family Relationships: A New Baby

Whether you plan it or not, another baby (or two) may show up in your family, and it could be sooner than you think. Another baby in the house can be a challenge when your twins are mere toddlers themselves! Our twins were 28 months of age when our fourth child was born—quite an adventure. I remember the hardest aspect of those initial months was trying to breastfeed our new baby. Our boys figured that when Mommy sat down to breastfeed the baby, they had the next 15 minutes to explore and wreak havoc—or so they thought. I had to get really creative to crack down on the madness so that I could continue to breastfeed our baby girl. Have interesting activities for your toddler twins hidden away, and pull them out at critical times when you're busy with your baby. You can use special crayons or a special rotating-toy basket that is brought out only during baby's feeding time, to be quickly stored away again when breastfeeding is complete so that it doesn't lose its appeal.

Although those early months were challenging, our twin boys were encouraged to mature with their baby sister's birth. Her presence in our family helped them grow up. Our twins were no longer the babies of our family! They were proud to show their sister how big kids do things. So if you find yourself pregnant again when your twins are still young, a lot of positives will result from the new family dynamic.

# Keeping a Twin-Friendly Budget: Saving Time and Money

When your twins are in the younger age-groups, borrow as many clothes for them from family and friends as you can, and shop your local Parents of Multiples club resales for gently used clothing. Let everyone know that you gladly accept hand-me-down clothes. Don't worry if some items have small stains. Save those pieces for home play days or as a change of pants during toilet training. Toddlers grow so fast that the borrowed items will soon be outgrown, and you'll be so glad you saved the money.

*Shoes* are an exception to the hand-me-down wardrobe. Every kid's feet are different (even identical twins), and every kid's walking pattern is slightly different, so brand-new shoes are preferable for molding to one's feet and being shaped by walking patterns. Personally, I have made it a point to ask family and friends for their kids' old clothes, and the money that I saved by not buying new pants and shirts was diverted into buying new shoes. We have found some trusty, comfortable, reliable sneaker brands that are our standby, day-to-day shoes. Add a slightly dressier shoe and you're pretty much set for any occasion. When at home, barefoot is best, but proper footwear is needed to venture outside.

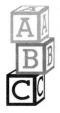

### Twin Tip

Try to buy your twins distinctive pairs of shoes; that way, each pair clearly belongs to a specific twin, and there is no squabbling over whose shoes are whose when rushing out the door. Using color themes for each child can extend to other items as well, such as drinking cups, to quickly identify whose cup is whose.

Your kids' shoes fit properly if there's a finger's breadth of distance from the tip of the toes to the tip of the insole. When our kids' feet grow, we use our favorite internet shoe store that has free shipping and free returns. We can confidently order the same brand and style of shoe, selecting a half size up, maybe getting new colors to be interesting. Because we know the shoe brand well, I am confident that the new shoe will fit. I spend mere minutes ordering online, and a couple of days later, the new shoes arrive on the doorstep. I found internet shopping to be much easier on our lifestyle than schlepping toddler twins to various shoe stores, looking for something you like and hoping that the store will have the size you need in stock.

Online shopping can be a real lifesaver. Many companies will offer free shipping if you pay more than a certain amount or will mail out special promotions for free shipping for a limited time. Be on the lookout for these offers. Try entering your favorite store's name with "coupon code" into your internet search engine to track down online shopping deals. You are too busy with 2 or more kids to be out shopping at brick-and-mortar stores.

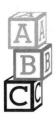

### Twin Tip

Figure out which internet shopping sites have good deals on shipping. Save time, effort, and gas money, and spend an afternoon having fun instead of shopping. Take a neighborhood walk, or hold a block-stacking competition! If you can streamline the mundane, routine, and yet necessary tasks such as shoe shopping for ever-growing feet, you can create more free time to enjoy your family.

# Having Fun

All children love to listen to music and dance. Music is such a great tension reliever for kids *and* parents, and it's a great alternative to flipping on the TV. Dance parties are an enjoyable way for toddler twins to let off energy and steam. Make sure you clear the floor of toys beforehand, as the dancing may get pretty wild! Excellent new kids' music that is family friendly *and* fun for adults to listen to is more popular these days than ever. I highly recommend They Might Be Giants albums specifically for kids, such as *Here Come the ABCs.*

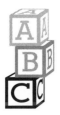

**Twin Tip**

Want to really have some fun with your toddler twins? Teach them "freeze dance," the classic game during which everyone must freeze like a statue when the music is paused. I guarantee a good time!

The music you play doesn't even have to be kids' music. Early Beatles albums are pretty kid friendly, for example. Make sure the music you listen to is fun for *all.* Your twins will notice when you really like a certain song and will enjoy hearing you sing along, even if you are off-key. Keep a stash of CDs in your car, or stock up your music selection on your smartphone for use with wireless communication to listen to good music while running errands and driving on longer car trips.

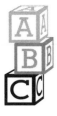

**Twin Tip**

Danielle, mom to school-aged twins, advises, "Enjoy the fact that your children have a built-in playmate."

Finally, part of having fun is keeping a healthy perspective on house-cleaning. Don't worry about a messy house. Within reason, let it go and play with your kids. Just make sure the floor isn't so cluttered that everyone's tripping everywhere. Your kids will not remember how clean the house was. They'll remember only the times that you played "fort" with them using couch cushions or when Dad played "garbage truck" with them by compacting them with throw pillows. Soon enough, your kids will grow older, and you can clean the house as much as you want. Reserve power clutter-busting sessions for the evenings when your kids are in bed, so that the floor actually stays clear for a while, and you and your partner can feel like normal people again, if for just a couple of hours.

CHAPTER 7

# The Preschool Years (3- and 4-Year-Olds)

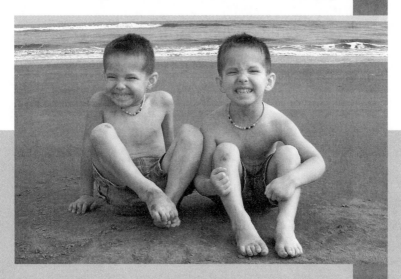

*M*ommy, can you come to my restaurant?" "Daddy, would you read this book to me?" All of a sudden, your twin babies have grown into 2 wonderful people who can speak clearly and play cooperatively with each other and others. The preschool years with twins are truly magical, as 3- and 4-year-olds burst with imagination. Not so long ago, your home was filled with constant feedings and frequent diaper changes. Now your home is a place where the couch is a train and a cardboard box is an airplane that you can fly to the grocery store to buy a loaf of bread.

 **Twin Tale**

Back in those hazy days when our twins were teeny, I never imagined that one day I'd hear this at our breakfast table.

**Andrew:** Knock, knock.

**Ryan:** Who's there?

**Andrew:** Rain.

**Ryan:** Rain who?

**Andrew:** Reindeer!

**Both:** Ba, ha, ha! (in that crazy way of laughing distinctive to a shared joke between twins)

Shared twin laughter is among the most beautiful things a parent can hear.

Relish these years and revel in playing like a child with your twins. Your preschool-aged children want nothing more than a parent sitting on the floor with them, following along in a make-believe scenario that they are creating as you go along. Be a customer in one child's restaurant and order a banana split with extra ketchup on top. Help your other child play "garbage truck" by collecting assorted toys and dumping them at a pretend garbage dump. Playtime serves a greater purpose than just fun. Through imaginative play, 3- and 4-year-olds make sense of the world around them.

The possibilities of imaginative scenarios are limitless with 2 kids at the same creative age. You have 2 inventive minds bouncing ideas off each other. And conveniently, you have multiple actors to play out different roles—store cashier and shopper, pilot and copilot, or waiter and customer, for example.

Your twins are most likely wonderful playmates much of the time. However, do not expect your twins to play wonderfully with each other all the time, every day. Could you imagine being with the same person *all the time*? Two individuals with 2 minds of their own will have differing opinions from time to time. Disagreements between your twins are inevitable.

Is there a way to prevent inter-twin arguments from happening? Not completely, but there *is* a way to reduce the number of disagreements in your home. Giving each child his own personal space is one way to prolong the peace in your home. If you respect the individual opinions and personal space of your children, each will feel more self-assured, secure, and content. In this way, you can prevent some arguments from even starting.

Parents of preschool-aged twins notice that life is much easier than it was a couple of years earlier because twins can be such great playmates. However, keep in mind that your twins won't want to play together all the time, despite the convenience of such an arrangement for you as a parent. Each child needs her own distinct relationships with other siblings, relatives, and friends—these relationships are all part of healthy and normal child development. These relationships help each child build her sense of identity and self-esteem. You'll notice different patterns emerging as, for example, one twin buddies up with an older sibling frequently one month, while the next month, your other twin takes great interest in a neighborhood friend. As a parent of twins, encourage these budding outside relationships. Your children will always have a unique and special twin bond, but early experiences with others help socialize each twin as she embarks on her school years. Such socialization is great for adjusting to a classroom setting. Much of the focus of the early school years is simply getting along with others and listening to instructions. Your twins will be well prepared for school simply by socializing with the world around them.

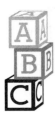

## Twin Tip

For the first couple of years, you synchronized your infant twins' schedules to make life more manageable. Now, at the preschool stage of the game, parenting twins is less about daily survival and more about nurturing the individuality of each child.

# Sleep Issues

On average, 3- and 4-year-olds should be sleeping a total of 12 hours in a 24-hour period. Your twins may have given up their naps or, if bedtime is later or they've woken up early, they may take a quick 1- to 2-hour early afternoon nap. Expect a few months' time of an in-between phase. Some days, your twins may need the nap, and other days, quiet time will suffice. As discussed in the previous chapter, encourage an hour of quiet time in the early afternoon (see the Need for Naps [or Quiet Time] section on pages 111–112 for more information on quiet time). A restful break from the day's activities helps your twins be energized for the remainder of the day. Be flexible and creative with naps. One twin may like to keep napping, while his twin doesn't need to. Allow one twin to nap in the shared bedroom while you read quietly with your other twin in your bedroom, for example.

If your twins share a bedroom, one twin may wake your other twin too early in the morning. Encourage both twins to stay in bed if the sun hasn't come up yet. They're old enough now to understand what you expect of them. For example, teach them that if one child wakes up and it's light outside but the other is still sleeping, the twin who is awake should quietly tiptoe out of the room so as not to disturb the other. You'll likely have several mornings where one twin is bright-eyed and bushy-tailed, while his twin is still yawning with heavy eyelids. If you don't all have to leave the house that morning, encourage your sleepy twin to go back to bed, making a teaching point for your awake twin so that he can learn for the next time.

A great way to help ensure a good night's sleep is to make sure your twins get plenty of activity and exercise during the daytime. Your preschoolers are naturally filled with energy! Getting lots of activity during the day will help your twins be more restful at night. Playgrounds help kids exercise their large muscle groups by climbing and balancing. Neighborhood and nature walks, with short bursts of running sprinkled throughout, get kids' legs moving. Get your twins practicing on tricycles, and advance to 12-inch bikes with training wheels once they're a bit taller. Don't forget the bike helmets! Make learning new physical activities fun. Simply running around the yard can provide great physical activity. Or you can play catch or "monkey in the middle."

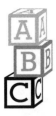

**Twin Tip**

Aim for at least 30 minutes a day of cumulative physical activity. The exercise still counts if it is done in smaller bursts scattered throughout the day, and it promotes better quality nighttime sleep.

In wintertime or during bad weather, you'll need to get creative to find ways to get your twins' bodies moving and hearts pumping. Clear out your play area for a safe game of catch with a soft ball, or play hide-and-seek. Our family cleared the space in our unfinished basement, cushioned wall corners and sharp edges, and kept our boys' bikes there all winter. Many afternoons, we'd head downstairs so that our boys could strap on their bike helmets and have a ball riding their bikes around while it was freezing cold outside. See what fun ideas you can come up with to squeeze in daily physical activity to help your twins sleep more solidly at night.

Sometimes, I'd be somewhat ridiculous and suggest we run around the house 2 or 3 times. I always remember Ryan, panting after his third round, asking me "Can I keep going?" "Sure!" I would reply. Years later, he runs distance with his school's cross-country team. I think it's funny that my goofy strategies those earlier years led to the discovery of his love for running later on.

## Socialization: Twins' Roles Within a Family

Your 3-year-old twins are eager to learn about the world around them. When kids have a strong sense of their roles within a family, self-esteem gets a boost and they more easily navigate through their lives, at all ages. How can a 3-year-old feel like part of a family? Enlist their help around the house. Taking care of the home is not just a parent's job. It is *every* family member's responsibility, and you can exercise the philosophy starting at a young age.

Preschool-aged kids *love* to help with housework. Give your twins dust cloths to clean off tabletops while you vacuum. Sorting laundry? Make a pile of your twins' clothes and have each child put the clean items back into the proper drawer. Teach your kids where everything goes so that they can help again the next time. Coaching your kids to perform simple housework tasks may seem like *more* work initially, but the rewards are worth the effort. Your

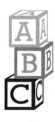

**Twin Tip**

Big-box stores often have nice-looking nonbreakable dinnerware (melamine as one example, usually intended for outdoor entertaining). Have a set on hand, and your twins can help set the table each night without fear of broken dishes. See the next chapter, specifically page 179 of the Age-Appropriate Chores for Kids section, for an age-appropriate chore chart.

twins will learn quickly, and soon you will see that they *really are* helping. Besides, daily mundane house chores are more fun when tackled as a team.

When your twins help with household chores, the job doesn't have to be performed perfectly. Applaud each child's *effort,* not the outcome. Chores help each twin feel like a contributing member of your family, which will go a long way to boosting his self-esteem. The bonus for you? A 3-year-old who is accustomed to helping around the house will grow into an older child who helps around the house. Expect each child to help at a young age so that it becomes a natural part of everyone's routine. Eight-year-olds won't magically start tidying up their bedrooms on their own without having had some prior experience.

The most important job your twins can help with is keeping the toy clutter under control. Multiple young children in a single home can quickly result in a crowded floor of random toys. Coach them to put away toys when they are finished playing with them. Big baskets and totes can simplify the process (eg, cars in one basket, trains in another, and stuffed animals in a third).

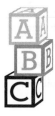

**Twin Tip**

Borrow an organization strategy from preschool teachers: take digital pictures of each toy group and print them. Tape the pictures to storage bins so that nonreaders can check the picture to see what goes where.

We're not looking for perfect organization from 3-year-olds. We're simply sending the broader message that when you're done playing with something, you should pick up after yourself. Make cleanup fun! Set an egg

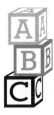

### Twin Tip

Organization in your twins' closet can streamline your morning routine. Choosing their own clothes to wear each day helps your twins feel as if they have some control over their daily lives. Organize your twins' clothing into groups of play clothes and nicer clothes. Depending on the day's activities, you can instruct your twins to dress themselves in play clothes, for example, if you are all headed to a neighborhood playground. Your children get a sense of ownership by having a choice, and they are still dressed appropriately for the occasion.

timer for 3 minutes and have a speedy cleanup race to see how much can be put away before the timer goes off. Once everyone gets into the habit of helping clean up, it becomes part of the daily routine.

Your twins will learn to interact with the outside world by getting lots of practice at home interacting with family members. Age-appropriate board or card games are a great way to teach social skills while getting in some good family bonding time. Your twins will learn to take turns and have fun whether they win or lose. They may have a hard time sitting still for longer stretches. If one runs off after only one turn, that's OK. Just continue the game with your other child as long as the players remaining are still having fun. If your first twin decides to come back, simply have him pick up where he left off.

When playing board games with my kids at this age, I rarely fully followed the included instructions. If no one wants to play anymore, don't sweat it. Pack up the game and try again another day. Expecting 3-year-olds to sit perfectly still through an entire board game is unrealistic. Over time and with practice, you will see that your young twins will be able to sit for longer stretches, they will be more cooperative during the game, and the games will be more meaningful for them (ie, there is more to it than just moving a red game piece around in a random circle). If one child wants to play a game with an older sibling, great! Encourage your twins to split up when they feel like it.

# Preparing for Preschool

The idea of your children spending a couple of hours in a classroom setting away from you and your partner, siblings, and possibly each other can be quite a change for everyone involved. If your twins have spent time in a child care setting, the transition may not be as dramatic as for those who have been cared for at home or in a smaller group setting. Our generation may or may not have attended preschool back when we were young. Today, however, education experts agree that the experience of a preschool program can help kids learn more effectively when kindergarten comes along. We're talking about a fun, relaxed preschool atmosphere, not any sort of rigorous academic curriculum. In preschool, 3-year-olds usually participate 2 or 3 half days a week, while 4-year-olds can participate 3 or 4 half days a week.

Preschool registration happens at different times depending on where you live. In general, for most areas, looking at preschool options a year before you plan on enrolling your twins is a good idea. Busy urban settings can be more competitive, and infants on preschool waiting lists are not uncommon in larger cities. Check with your local park district for good options, and talk with your neighbors who have older kids to see whether they liked their private preschool. If your children were born preterm or needed early intervention therapy services (eg, speech therapy) before 3 years of age, they may qualify for preschool through your school district. Contact your local public school district to get specifics on requirements for qualification.

 **Twin Tale**

Once upon a time, I took our twin boys, recently turned 3 years of age, to a library story hour. After about 5 minutes, both boys started wandering around the room instead of sitting quietly to listen. I gathered them together in the back of the room and told them, just one time, "Let's try to sit and listen. If you can't sit and listen, we'll have to leave so we don't disturb the other kids." That day, our boys just weren't interested. I wanted them to appreciate these sorts of experiences and to have positive associations with them, not to remember their mom nagging them for 30 minutes. So I simply gathered our boys up and we left. No sense in forcing the issue—this is supposed to be *fun* for your kids. Just try again another day. Keep exposing your twins to the idea of story hour and similar experiences, and they'll learn to appreciate them.

In the months leading up to preschool, you'll want to provide your twins with some practice for the experience. Look around your community for options. Public libraries or bookstores usually offer a story hour or craft sessions for each young age-group. These story hours are a great way for your twins to practice sitting quietly in a group while listening to a story. That these programs are usually free is a bonus. Your twins will learn some social etiquette by being in a room of 3-year-olds. Multiples may be accustomed to close physical contact with each other, but they'll need to learn they can't be quite so cozy with others around them.

Another way to get your twins ready for preschool is to visit your area's public and school playgrounds after school hours. Get to know a variety of parks around your home to keep the trips interesting. Your kids will have fun on different types of equipment and feel quite comfortable at their preschool playground when the time comes. Your twins will also gain a little experience meeting and playing with other kids at the playground.

Look into your local park district youth offerings and recreational youth sports. Always ask whether they offer a twins discount! Soccer is a great gender-neutral choice that boy-girl twins would enjoy. Park districts often offer a 3-year-old playgroup class, specifically for parents to drop their child off so that their child gets used to the idea of being on his own for a bit. To ease the transition, if your twins are in the same class, they can provide

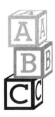

## Twin Tip

When your twins attend preschool, they will bring home mountains of adorable craft projects and paintings. The artwork and drawings of 2 students can quickly accumulate and overwhelm a home. How can you preserve the highlights of your kids' projects while minimizing clutter? Take digital photos of each child *individually* holding her artistic creation(s). You'll have documentation of the art and what your child looked like when she created the art, without taking up physical space on a shelf. Your twins will beam with pride when showing off their creation. After taking a digital picture, you can even hang the artwork in an art gallery on your twins' bedroom wall by using blue painter's tape. The tape can be rearranged multiple times without damaging painted walls or woodwork. An art gallery of preschool projects is a great way to boost your twins' self-esteem and encourage future projects. If the projects get crumpled or thrown out, no worries, because you've saved the projects with your digital camera.

some comfort for each other when you leave. At these types of classes, my twin boys were so excited to see new toys to play with that they didn't mind at all that Mom was leaving for a while. I had tears myself, though, the first couple of times and didn't know whether I felt better or I felt worse that my boys weren't crying at these goodbyes. With a little practice getting out there with your twins, you'll all be ready to make the leap to 2 mornings a week of preschool quite smoothly.

Many parents of twins wonder whether they should keep them in the same classroom for preschool or separate them into different classrooms. If your preschool is a small program, you may have no choice because all the 3-year-olds are together in a single class. If there are 2 separate classrooms, you'll have to decide for your family on the best strategy. Remember that this decision is not final. Every year, you can (and should) reassess your family's situation to determine what classroom placement will work best for your twins for the new school year.

 **Twin Tale**

Sue, mom to third-grade twins, advises, "It is OK to separate twins into 2 classrooms. They will still feel connected. Also, don't worry if they are progressing at different stages."

For our family's situation, our decision for class placement was pretty straightforward. We felt that our identical twin sons looked so similar that the teachers and other students would be confused all year long as to who each twin was. We didn't want our sons to hear the question "Which one are you?" all the time. I wanted to de-emphasize my boys' "twinness" and give my boys a chance to show others who they are as a person, as an individual. I also felt that 2 mornings a week of being in 2 separate classrooms wouldn't be that big of a deal, considering my boys are together the other 5 days a week, 24 hours a day. In addition, I felt that after some practice with separate preschool classrooms, the transition into separate classrooms in the higher grades would be a little easier.

The issue of twin placement in classrooms is a big issue, as many families feel that their kids would do better in school if their twins were in the same classroom. These families argue that they, not the school, should make the final decision of class placement. New legislation has been popping up

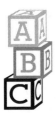

**Twin Tip**

If your twins are in 2 separate classrooms in school, prepare in advance for special school days such as Meet the Teacher Day. Arrange for both parents to attend or have Grandma or another trusted adult help on the special day. Let the teachers know your situation in advance and that you plan on spending time in both classrooms to see both kids and both environments. If only one parent can attend, explain the situation to the teachers so that they can fill you in on important information that you may have missed while moving between the 2 classes.

in various states, giving families the final say in whether twins are placed together or separately. Each family must assess its own situation and decide what will work best for its particular situation. Some families find that keeping twins together in the early years helps smooth the way for eventual separation in the higher grades.

 **Twin Tale**

Michelle, mom to identical boys in third-grade, recalls, "I recommend flexibility and using your best judgment. I had so much pressure to separate my boys, so I did, but they were not ready and melted down. We kept them together until third grade, at which time we felt they were ready to separate. They are now doing great! Each boy has different likes and needs, and I accommodate them as 2 individual people."

Parents can observe the classroom dynamic, meet classmates, get to know the teacher better, make their child feel special, and help out the school all in the matter of a couple of hours by volunteering in their child's classroom. Preschools usually love parents' hands-on involvement in the classroom, and kids get a real ego boost in showing off their class and parents to each other. My kids' school experiences were somewhat of a mystery to me until I spent some time assisting in the classroom. After you spend a little time with the class, you'll be able to ask each child specific questions about friends or workstations because you've seen the class in action firsthand. Even if you work outside the home, I recommend arranging for a morning off from work to spend an hour or so with the class. If your twins are in 2 separate classrooms, be sure to post your volunteer dates prominently on your family calendar, and talk about the timing with your kids to prevent any jealousy or concerns about fairness.

## One-on-one Time

Continue to carve out as much one-on-one time as you can with each of your twins during their preschool years. Recognizing and stealing moments of time throughout a regular day is a good strategy. Read with one twin while your other is playing with airplanes, for example. Continue to take just one child, alone, on outings with you when another parent or adult can help out.

We've taken one-on-one time to a new level in our family with special airplane trips with Mom. We have extended family scattered around the country and have found airfare for 2 family members much more affordable than for the whole family of 6. We can reduce traveling costs, visit faraway family, and squeeze in special time with each child, all at once. We rotate these trips through the birth order to be fair to all 4 of our kids. These special trips are such a treat for our kids, and I always come away from each experience with a new appreciation for who each of my children is as an individual.

## Two Distinct Individuals

Whenever I meet someone who happened to grow up as a twin, I always ask if there was anything he would have preferred his parents to have done differently. Most of the time, the response I hear is some variation on a similar theme: I wish our parents didn't..."give us the same thing for our birthday," "dress us in identical outfits," or "expect us to share everything."

While some people assume all twins are the same, others take it to the other extreme. Many people ask me whether my twin sons are opposites. Is one social, while your other is a recluse? Is one more talkative and your other quiet? Or, my favorite, "Which is the good one?" These questions imply that each twin's character traits are defined as the opposite of those of his twin brother. Of course, this is not the case; they are individuals, and each child is complete on his own.

Any individual can be like another in some respects and different in other ways. Everybody, whether born as a twin or not, desires to be treated as an individual. Parents of all twins, identical or same-sex fraternal twins more so, need to think about this daily. You're a busy parent, and it may be quicker or more efficient at times to treat your twins as a unit, but I encourage you to treat your twins as siblings who happen to have been born on the same day.

A great way to encourage individuality is to read their bedtime stories to them separately at night. When our twin boys were babies and toddlers, we were operating in survival mode, so we usually read to them simultaneously. As the years progressed, and our twins were easier to care for, we saw that it would benefit both boys to have their bedtime stories read to them one-on-one. Reading to each twin separately boosts early reading skills and creates a calmer atmosphere in which to quiet down and settle in with a good book. The time and work to read to your twins individually is well worth the effort. Your twins won't distract each other and will get a lot more out of the experience. Try to alternate which twin reads with which parent each night. Be realistic, though, and on late nights, or if one parent is handling bedtime solo, gather everyone to snuggle up for the bedtime stories.

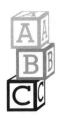

**Twin Tip**

My identical twins didn't quite realize that they were different from other kids until their preschool years. All of a sudden, they realized that not everyone else has an identical-looking sibling the same age! Whenever someone would ask one of my twins, "Which one are you?" he would look at the person with bemused disbelief. If your twins are the same sex, dress them in different clothing to help friends and classmates know who is who. If your twins look a great deal alike, *talk* about it with them. They are so used to life with a twin that they may not realize that others can't tell them apart. You can even role-play social situations. Teach your twins to introduce themselves clearly, and teach each child how to politely correct someone who has guessed his identity incorrectly.

Multiples know how to share well, having shared their parents with each other since they were newborns, but expecting them to share *all* their things, *all* the time, is unrealistic. You'll want to have a system to give each child her own personal space. Even if your twins share a bedroom, you can provide each one with a distinctly colored box, or even her own shelving unit (safely strapped to the wall to prevent falls, of course), that she can keep her special things in—a rock collection, a party favor from a friend's birthday, or whatever she decides is important to her.

 **Twin Tale**

Bonnie, an adult identical twin, states, "While I appreciate everything my parents did for me while I was growing up, there are several things that I would do differently if I had twins or I would suggest to those who have twins. Growing up, my mom dressed my sister and me the same until about seventh grade. Looking back, I kind of wish she would have let us dress in our own style. We were in the same class in school until we were in high school. Unfortunately, we went to a small school, so there wasn't a choice, but this led us to have the same friends until high school."

Remind each twin to respect her sibling's personal space—older and younger siblings' spaces as well, as twins can outnumber an older sibling and confiscate a toy by sheer manpower alone. Give each twin her own distinct-looking piggy bank to collect loose coins. Institute a house rule that you can check only your own piggy bank's contents.

In your living and play areas, create separate play stations so that there are interesting things to do at different places in the home. One twin can play board games in one area, while your other goes in another room to look at books. Don't expect your twins to play with the same items all the time. Give each child some space and breathing space, and your days will be more harmonious.

On birthdays and holidays, give each child distinctive presents. At 3 and 4 years of age, each child has particular interests. Pick up on these differences and use them as inspiration for giving separate gifts. Adult twins groan when they remember all the times they received 2 of the same item. When our twins were 3 years of age, we noticed that sharks fascinated Ryan and that Andrew was interested in fire trucks, so on their birthday, we ran with these themes. Emphasize to family members to look for distinctive gifts for your twins. They'll likely appreciate a little coaching, so help them out with ideas.

If your twins are identical or of the same sex and fraternal, it is inevitable that friends and family will occasionally be stumped—who is who? Every week at my identical twin sons' preschool, a friend or teacher would mistake each boy for his twin brother. Such confusion becomes a part of life, a routine, and each twin gets plenty of practice reminding people who he is.

On one special day each year, however, twins should not have to repeatedly remind others of who they are—their birthday. When my twins turned 5, we threw a big party, inviting friends and classmates from both boys' classrooms. I wanted to minimize any confusion over each twin's identity. I found a great online website that lets you customize T-shirts any way you choose. Each boy wore distinctly colored T-shirts at the birthday celebration with his name printed on the front and back, as well as "It's my birthday!" on the front (I added that because I figured classmates' parents would not necessarily know who the birthday kids were).

All toys that enter your home will eventually get shared extensively. After all, playing with all the cumulative toys, rather than just your own portion, is more fun. But initially, on gift-giving occasions, give each child at least a day or so with his new toy before he is expected to share with others. After the first couple of days, or a period that seems appropriate, the new items can become part of the public domain, fair game for all.

If your twins are squabbling over who gets to play with a new item, after a certain amount of time, use the egg timer trick. Give each child a timed turn with the toy, and rotate turns. The egg timer helps reassure your twins that the turns will be fair.

## Expanding Social Circles

For several years, our boys were in 2 separate classes in school, and usually a classmate would invite just our boy who was in the same class to his birthday party—this is a *good* thing. Attending a friend's party without one's twin is a great learning opportunity.

Starting as early as the preschool years, social experiences independent of one's twin will help each child gain confidence as an individual. My twins are identical, and often in social situations when both boys are present, a lot of time is spent answering the question "Which one are you?" I have observed that when one boy has a chance to play or hang out with friends on his own, more time is spent in meaningful interaction rather than clarifying his identity.

If one of your twins tends to be shy without the nearby presence of his twin, the experience can be especially beneficial to his emotional maturity.

Preschool parties are usually just a couple of hours, anyway—a brief and fun way to practice being on one's own.

I have heard of instances when only one twin is invited to a party and his parents ask whether they can bring along their other twin as well. I recommend against this practice. Yes, it requires more effort to arrange for trustworthy child care for your other kid(s), but it is well worth the effort for your invited child to have the party experience solo.

Are you concerned that your other twin will get jealous? Kids are resilient, and the experiences will even out over time. Matter-of-factly explain, for example, "Today, it is John's turn to go to a party. Soon it will be Joseph's turn." Kids follow their parents' emotional cues. If you are calm and matter-of-fact about the situation, your children will be as well. Plus, you can provide the non-partying twin with special time as well (such as a trip to a playground)—a win-win situation for everybody.

## Consistency and Discipline

By the time your twins are 3 and 4 years of age, they should have a clear understanding of what the house rules are and a sense of what is appropriate behavior. Hopefully, you've been able to lay down a consistent framework of rules in your twins' toddler years on which you can continue to build. High expectations of your twins' behavior from an early age have a lot of benefits. Instead of having to undo a year's worth of poor behavior, you are providing positive reinforcement for appropriate behavior.

While more mature than toddlers, 3- and 4-year-olds are still growing and learning and will continue to test limits and rules. The testing of limits is age-appropriate behavior and not a deliberate attempt on your twins' part to drive you crazy! Your kids will test you in different situations to see whether the rules still hold water. Your twins are also meeting new friends at school and recreation programs who behave in different ways, and they will wonder whether they can try out some of those new behaviors at home with you. You need to hold strong and be consistent with your house rules.

If your child disobeys a rule, don't give endless warnings with no consequences; give a *time-out*. Remember that a proper time-out takes place in a boring location for 1 minute for each year of your child's age (ie, 3 or 4 minutes for preschoolers). (For more on discipline, read the previous chapter, specifically the Kind and Effective Discipline section on pages 120–125.)

When time is up, tell your child briefly what she did wrong, have her apologize to the appropriate person if the situation calls for it, and move on with your day. Don't dwell on the misbehavior or give it undue attention. You don't want to reward poor behavior with extra attention.

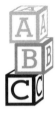

## Twin Tip

You do not need to give each of your twins separate warnings about the same issue when they are *both* present for the original warning. Let your twins know, "When I say something to one of you, I am saying it to both of you." If you use this consistent pattern to deal with twins' misbehavior, you'll save a lot of time and energy down the line by preventing your kids from experimenting to find different parental responses.

## Balancing the Social Dynamic

You may notice a new phenomenon in your home now that your twins are preschool aged—teaming up against other siblings or friends. By this age, they have a tight bond with each other and consider each other teammates of sorts. Be aware that your twins may, perhaps unwittingly, gang up on others. Nip this sort of behavior in the bud. Explain to your twins that you expect them to be kind to and share with *all* their siblings, not just their twin.

Preschool-aged twins may preferentially share things with each other yet instantly become territorial if their older or younger sibling shows interest—the tight twin bond illustrating itself once again. Monitor these situations to make sure their single-born siblings aren't getting railroaded or just passively allowing certain situations to keep the peace. This is a form of bullying, and it shouldn't be tolerated.

Don't forget, as discussed in the Kind and Effective Discipline section on pages 120 to 125 in the previous chapter, you should avoid asking, "Who started it?" A fight takes 2 kids, and if you ask who started it, your twins will learn to manipulate your reactions. You want them to learn how to settle their differences on their own, without an ever-present parent mediator, not how to pin the blame on their twin.

## Expectations on Outings

As your twins grow older, you're probably going on more family outings to museums, zoos, or parks. New situations run more smoothly if you remind your twins what you expect of their behavior *beforehand*. When you get to the zoo, before everyone unbuckles to get out of the car, take a moment to talk with your kids about what you expect. Remind them, for instance, "The zoo can be a busy place and there are lots of cool things to see, but everyone has to *stay together as a group*. Don't just run off if you see the giraffe! Tell Dad you want to see the giraffes and we'll all go together." Your kids will be reminded to use their self-control, and you won't lose them in a crowd of strangers. Give your kids lots of practice and they'll learn with repeated outings.

Anticipatory talks before new situations can help your kids remember how to behave. These talks are a kind and gentle way to lay out expectations that you can draw on if someone behaves poorly. If you're all going to have to wait in line at the store, remind your twins beforehand that you expect them to stand quietly with you and not run around loudly. If you are going to a friend's house for lunch, remind everyone of proper behavior before you get out of the car.

When my 4 kids were quite young, I took them to museums and zoos by myself numerous times. I suppose I wasn't truly by myself—I had my 4 kids with me! We've had some great adventures, my kids learned a lot, and the trips boosted my confidence as a parent. I always received comments from other parents, though, who were apparently shocked that my kids weren't running away from me. I've heard, "I don't know how you do it alone. I couldn't because my kid's a runner," many times.

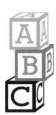

### Twin Tip

How can you keep your kids together as a group during an outing? Again, before getting out of the car, remind everyone of the rule of staying as a group. Then, during the outing, if one of your kids runs off, she should temporarily lose the privilege of walking independently "like a big kid." She should hold your hand or hold on to the stroller (if you're using one for a younger sibling) for the next 10 minutes, and if she is well-behaved, she can earn back the privilege of walking *with the group*.

If one or more of your kids are not getting the message and are repeatedly running off, you'll have to cut the outing short, explaining to your kids that because they can't follow the rules, they cannot stay and have fun. Cutting a zoo trip short if someone's misbehaving is unpleasant, but letting your kids know that behaving properly and staying with the group is more important.

## When Twins Collide

Twins are extremely close, yet when they fight, look out! Twins' fights can be more extreme and emotional than fights between other siblings precisely because they are so close. Feelings are hurt more deeply when a stronger connection exists.

How can you reduce the amount of infighting among your multiples? Look for frequent trouble spots and figure out solutions. In our family, car safety seat location was quite a hot topic. After a particularly bad week, filled with fights over who got to sit in which car safety seat, I had to lay down the law. We would alternate between 2 car safety seats monthly. Andrew would sit in the preferred seat during September, for example, and Ryan would sit in that seat during October. Everyone knew what to expect, and our kids knew we wouldn't waffle, so they didn't bother trying to change the system. The bonus of this system is that your kids learn the months of the year. Perhaps your twins both desire the same chair at the dinner table. If your twins are having repeated arguments over the same issue, strategize to see whether a new system can promote peace.

## Interactions With Other Siblings

Be aware of the dynamic between your twins and their other siblings, whether older or younger. Patrick, 12-year-old brother to 10-year-old twin girls, notes that "sometimes they gang up on you." My singleton children would agree with this statement. It is somewhat inevitable with the team-like nature of the twin bond, but it is something for parents to be aware of. It is also a reason to promote one-on-one time, and make sure you experiment with different groupings of your kids. For example, bring only one twin and your oldest singleton with you on a Saturday to run errands, leaving your other twin at home with your partner.

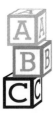

## Twin Tip

An environment rich with words will help boost your children's language development. Even the busiest of parents can use everyday time with their kids to narrate out loud what is happening in their daily lives. You may feel a bit like a news reporter, but even mundane tasks such as preparing the morning breakfast can be a speech-boosting session. Turn off the TV, turn your cell phone to vibrate and put it away, and focus on your kids. Simply being *present* and communicative with your children will go a long way toward boosting their future speech and cognitive skills. For further advice on boosting your kids' language development, visit the official American Academy of Pediatrics website for parents, HealthyChildren.org.

# Advanced Toilet Training and Independence

Do not despair if your twins are not fully toilet-trained by their third birthday. Continue to be as patient and supportive as you can be, which is easier said than done. Toileting accidents (wetting or soiling) can be extremely frustrating, more so for us parents of multiples and more so if your kids have been training for a while. After their third birthday, toilet training can take on a new dimension. A 3-year-old can be more stubborn than a 2-year-old and is more likely to dig her heels in if there is a battle of wills.

Power struggles can be more frequent and severe than in the past. As a parent, you need to relax as best you can, as frustrating as the situation may be. If you get more emotional and upset with your twins, they may resist toileting even more as a result. At the preschool age, a child truly has a mind of her own, and ultimately, she has to decide for herself to toilet on her own.

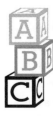

## Twin Tip

Sometimes one twin may backtrack and start having toileting accidents (wetting or soiling) and as a result get more attention during cleanup, as well as lectures. Be careful of paying one twin too much attention for accidents. His twin may start to also have accidents in a subconscious attempt to get some additional attention.

If you have a difficult week filled with accidents, you may have to stop for a while. Make sure your twins help clean up their pee or poop (in an age-appropriate way), and have them get their own fresh clothes to help them realize how much easier it is to pee and poop into the toilet, not into the underwear.

Use success sticker charts in the case of toileting regression. You can make the charts as specific as you like. If only one twin is having poop accidents, for example, create just one poop chart for her to help her get back on track.

True toilet training is complete when your twins do not need reminders to use the toilet. When you notice that they've been doing well with parental reminders, back off a bit and see whether they remind themselves. The sooner your kids learn to remind themselves to use the toilet, the more independent they will be. If you require further assistance with toilet training, or your twins are having problems such as constipation, consult with your pediatrician.

A friend with triplets had a challenge when her kids were 3½. While 2 of her kids were happily and successfully using the potty, her remaining daughter, despite prior successes, refused the potty in a classic display of 3-year-old power. Toilet training is a whole new ball game once a child is older than 3 years.

Three-year-old kids are smart, have a better sense of how the world works, and continue to realize that their actions have an effect on their caregivers and environment. Twenty-four–month-old kids are no strangers to the concept of power struggles, but it is quite different to deal with a 3½-year-old's efforts to assert her independence and control over her own body. As always, every child is different, and you know your kids best. If you have specific concerns about your child, or are worried about underlying problems, consult with your pediatrician.

All too often, toilet-training advice found in books and parenting magazines can be geared toward situations in which a caregiver and child are one-on-one in some sort of magical bubble, with no interference from the real world, family and work schedules, or even siblings. Most of us live in homes full of little people and action. For any family, but especially when training twins or more, many factors are at play that can have a big effect on the progress of training.

Ultimately, a 3-year-old is in control of her own body, and she needs to be the one making the decision to toilet properly. She cannot be forced (the phrase "You can lead a horse to water..." comes to mind). There is no quick, overnight fix. Toilet training is a process. But parents of 3-year-olds should remove the use of disposable pull-up pants during daytime hours. Many mistakenly think of pull-up pants as cloth training pants. But let's be honest—they are simply a disposable, absorbent diaper in pull-up pants form. And too often they prolong the course of a child's learning to use the toilet because they are an out. Your child doesn't need to run to the toilet when she feels the natural sensations to pee or poop, and she can simply do the deed in the convenience of the pull-up pants she is already wearing. That said, pull-up pants for overnight sleep, until nighttime dryness is consistent, is perfectly fine.

The ultimate goal is for your child to wear clean, dry underwear. To reach that goal, your child needs practice wearing actual cotton underwear during increasing stretches of time over the course of a day. She will learn what happens if she does not make it to the potty in time. Yes, this means accidents for 2 or more kids. But mistakes are a part of life and are part of the learning process. Your child should also be sitting on the toilet or potty seat at regular times each day, regardless of result (eg, first thing in the morning, after lunch).

Parents of twins can preserve some sanity by having systems in place to simplify cleaning up the inevitable pee and poop. Three-year-olds are developmentally ready to become active participants in self-care, so they can (and should) help when accidents occur. When a child is an active helper with accidents, she'll see that peeing and pooping into the toilet is much simpler (and more rewarding with positive reinforcement) than all the cleanup. Whenever a child has an accident, caregivers should be matter-of-fact (more on this later) and direct their child straight to the potty. "Oops, you need to pee. Let's go to the potty." Even if nothing else will come out, you need to help your child make the connection that the sensation of needing to pee or poop is associated with sitting on the toilet. After your child has been sitting on the toilet for a bit, help remove the wet or soiled clothing, and have your child take the wet clothing to the laundry area herself. To minimize stress over laundry, we used to keep a bucket in our utility sink in the laundry area to streamline the eventual laundering. Place a kid-friendly step stool in front to help your 3-year-old reach the bucket.

Then your child should be the one to get fresh underwear and clothes and put them on.

When toilet training all 4 of our kids, we kept a huge stack of absorbable cloths (repurposed old burp cloths from the baby days) handy in a cabinet in a central location of our home. An adult caregiver will perform the bulk of the real cleaning of the floor (eg, wet-dry vacuum), but the child should go get a couple cloths from the stack, come help clean the mess (meaning an honest, 3-year-old effort), and bring the dirty cloths to the laundry bucket to be dealt with later.

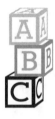

**Twin Tip**

When you deal with the inevitable toileting accidents (wetting or soiling), you may feel angry and frustrated, but do your best to keep your cool. Even negative attention is attention, and when you have children who share a caregiver most of the time, the desire for attention can complicate matters.

Throughout the toilet-training process, be mindful of your language. Many of us instinctively say, "Don't you want to pee on the potty like a big kid?" However, coaxing your child with this phrase is not always helpful. To a 3-year-old, the idea of being a big kid, with all the added expectations and responsibilities, may not sound so desirable. Your 3-year-old may think that life as a baby, with the cuddling and oodles of caregiver attention, sounds like a pretty good arrangement, thank you very much.

An additional note about pull-up pants, specifically during nap time, child care, or preschool hours: talk with your child care providers to make sure everyone is on the same page. Preschools often ask for pull-up pants during school hours; however, this can complicate matters. Some kids save their daily poop for that 2-hour stretch when they know they're going to wear pull-up pants. Similarly, many kids older than 3 years who wear pull-up pants for naps may poop specifically at nap time. Depending on your child's age and progress, talk with your child's caregivers at school, and work together toward a plan. A 2-week winter break without travel plans would be an example of a good time to focus on wearing normal underwear for increasing stretches of time without any interruptions from a school schedule. Ultimately, map out a timeline for raising the bar for your child to rise to the occasion and make good progress.

# Emotional and Social Support for Parents

Your day-to-day routine with your twins is much easier than in the past, but it's still a lot of work. Parents of young children need to seek out ways to relieve the stress and laugh about the current craziness of their lives. A positive mental attitude goes a long way in helping you survive the chaos of each day. Spilled milk? Kids not listening the fifth time you've told them something? The next time you feel yourself losing your temper, try to see the humor in the situation.

Is splashed bathwater all over the bathroom floor? Have your crew grab towels with you and mop it up, telling them, "Well, this is one way to get the floor clean!" Lots of mishaps can occur each day. Life is more fun if you can laugh about it and move on.

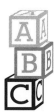

## Twin Tip

Some days you may feel as if you're telling your preschoolers the same things 100 times! Use humor so that you don't lose your cool. Your twins learn how to handle tense situations by watching you. When one of my then 4-year-old twins was not listening to me one evening, I wondered aloud, "Can we buy Andrew some new ears at the Ear Store? I think his are broken—he's not listening to his mom!" Andrew knew I was being goofy (not sarcastic; there's a big difference), and amidst the giggling, he understood that I was trying to get his attention. I had made my point in a fun way, not in a nagging, unpleasant way. And once I got him laughing, he was a lot more receptive to what I was saying.

Parenthood can be a tough road, but having comrades with you helps. Now that your twins are participating in more activities and attending preschool, you have a lot more opportunities to meet other parents of similar-aged kids. Reach out to make new acquaintances. Sharing stories and seeing that some of the struggles in your home are happening in other homes as well is very therapeutic. Parents share many of the same issues, whether or not they have twins. You can laugh about the struggles, remembering that each phase will pass quickly. If you're a naturally shy person, practice making small talk with other parents at a public park. Even if small talk doesn't lead to a lifelong friendship, it boosts your mood and takes you out of your own world.

---

 **Twin Tale**

Enjoy that you have the interesting family dynamic of multiples. Sheri, mom to preschool twins, shares, "My son Evan is always perplexed when he sees only one baby with a mommy and always asks where the other baby is." What an interesting perspective!

---

When out around town running errands, our family saw that the comments from strangers about our twins did not slow down. If anything, having a fourth child close in age increased the amount of comments we received. Far and away, the most common comment is "You've sure got your hands full!" Sometimes this line is delivered in a pitying tone with some headshaking, as if to say, "Wow, poor you!" Don't let these comments get under your skin. I am so used to hearing this phrase by now that I am ready with my reply: "They're good kids, and we're so lucky."

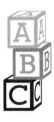 **Twin Tip**

As your twins grow older, keep trying your best to attend your local Parents of Multiples club meetings, even if you attend only once in a while. At a minimum, join their social media pages so that you've got interaction online and a forum to ask questions and seek support. You may feel that you've outgrown these meetings because you've moved past the newborn period, but if you can give another new parent of multiples some baby advice that you've lived and learned, you can see how far you've come on your parenting journey now that your twins are older. That can be quite a confidence builder, which can keep your spirits up.

View the interactions with interested strangers from your children's point of view. What should my twin sons think when we go out in public and people seem to feel sorry for their mom because of *them*? I never want my twins to feel that they are a burden on me. Even though I am talking with the stranger and not my kids, I want to send the message to my twins *every day* that they are loved, wanted, and wonderful.

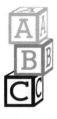

**Twin Tip**

I find that interactions with inquisitive, curious strangers can be a helpful way to boost my twins' self-esteem by complimenting them to others. An overheard compliment can be a lot more effective than simply telling your kids directly, "You are good kids and I love you."

# Budgeting and Practical Matters

Parenthood can be expensive, even with just one child. Twins need many of the same things at the same time and, therefore, can seem much costlier. When you're providing toys and experiences for your twins, remember that cost does not determine quality. Preschool-aged children can have a grand time with an empty cardboard box, which can be whatever they imagine it to be—a spaceship, a train, a house, or whatever your twins are in the mood for. The less a toy does, the more your kids think.

"Grocery store" and "restaurant" were 2 of our all-time favorite games to play at these ages. Save empty food containers such as butter tubs and cake mix boxes, clean them out, and use them as your groceries. You don't even need a toy play kitchen. You can create one out of an empty box by drawing a range on top with markers and decorating it however you please.

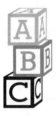

**Twin Tip**

Don't blow the bank buying toys for your twins. Think outside the box for interesting playthings. I found tailor's measuring tape at a craft store for a dollar, and my kids spent an afternoon measuring everything around the house. In fact, the first time I heard my son Ryan count to 50 was when he measured my bathroom countertop with the measuring tape. Some of the best toys don't have to be toys at all.

The public library can be a parent of multiples' best friend for sticking to a budget. Make a point to visit the library as much as you can to treat your twins. Let each child pick out his own book or more to give him a sense of ownership over the book. Having plenty of books available in your home will encourage your twins to become lifelong readers.

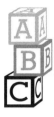

### Twin Tip

A bonus to museum and zoo memberships is that it is easier to plan spontaneous outings. Busy parents of twins don't have lots of extra time to research and explore countless options for a day trip. With a museum or zoo membership, you can take your family out without having to think or plan too hard. Once you've made a museum trip a couple of times, you'll really get to know the lay of the land. Bring your lunch along and you've got an affordable family day.

Budgeting for a family vacation is difficult when your family has 4 or more people. Airfare can be quite steep, especially because airlines charge kids older than 2 years the same fares as adults. You can take more vacations in your local area by considering family memberships to your area zoos and museums. Memberships are quite cost-effective for larger families and often pay for themselves in fewer than 2 visits a year. When you use a family membership, you don't feel pressured to see all the exhibits in one day. If one of your kids is cranky, you can leave early. We like having local memberships so that when the weather is nice, we can go to the zoo, and during hot or snowy seasons, we can go to the indoor aquarium.

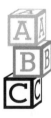

### Twin Tip

When you take your preschooler twins on outings, keep a stash of sandwich-sized plastic bags with your supplies. Distribute a healthy snack, such as clementine sections or apple slices, during the outing by handing out individual bags to each child—a more cost-effective method than purchasing convenience-sized packages (which usually contain processed, unhealthy options) at the store.

Another way to have some affordable family bonding time is with family movie picnics. Spread out some blankets in your family room, pop some popcorn, and play an age-appropriate movie or video. Let the cuddling and bonding commence! These picnics cost hardly anything and can be so much fun for all of you.

# Rainy Days: Painting for a Crowd

"Mom, can we paint?"

Even 1-year-olds can scribble and paint. It is a great way to boost hand and finger (fine motor) skills, feel the sensation of paint underneath fingertips, and just have some fun. Even older babies like to practice painting with pureed food on their high chair tray. As toddlers grow into preschoolers and beyond, the artwork matures into more significant forms and meaning, and painting, whether with fingers or brushes, is a great way to spend some time on a rainy or snowy day.

As a busy parent with 2 or more kids, though, you may sigh inwardly as you visualize 20 minutes of prep time, 2 minutes of painting, more paint on your children than the paper, and, inevitably, the painting cleanup. Our 4 kids loved painting when preschoolers, so we needed a system to make it easier on everyone.

An old mattress pad easily covers the kitchen table quickly and soaks up paint spills. Old pillowcases cover the chair backs for when kids get squirmy and lean over to check the progress of their siblings' projects. Old adult-sized T-shirts provide great art smock coverage, fastened in the back of the neck with a clip. The supplies can be stashed in one of those plastic zippered storage bags that new mattress pads come in at the store. Everything is stored together, easy to pull out and set up quickly.

When your Picassos and Monets are finished, simply pile up all the messy smocks and pillowcases in the center of the mattress pad, pull up the corners, and make a tidy, little bundle. All the messy stuff is safely contained within, and you can put the bundle into the laundry area and wash it when you have the time. Any washable paint-laden brushes can soak in the sink and be dealt with later.

The choices in washable paints and markers these days are dizzying. Kids don't even need fresh paper. Painting on old cardboard boxes or paper rescued from the recycling pile is just as fun. See what streamlining systems you can develop for your family so that cleanup after a fun time is a breeze.

# Enjoying the Here and Now

Savor playtime with your preschooler twins. Enjoy the fruits of your labor over the past 4 years. You've put so much effort and energy into your kids, and now you can relax a bit and enjoy these wonderful people that you have nurtured and guided. Don't be in a rush for the next stage of life. Play an extra board or card game with your twins, and enjoy this magical stage of their lives.

CHAPTER 8

# The School Years: As Your Twins Grow

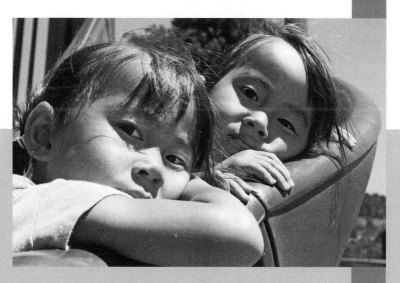

*O*ur twin sons, as preschoolers, loved to accompany their big brother to the bus stop on school mornings. One morning happened to be garbage and recycling pickup day. After the big kids' bus zoomed away to school, we returned to our home to see 2 large, now empty bins sitting at the end of the driveway. Without hesitation, Ryan and Andrew each grabbed one of the wheeled containers and began to roll the behemoths (relative to their small bodies) back into our garage. The bins towered well over their heads, and I called out, "That's OK, guys, I can get those!"

They quickly replied, "Mom, we're strong; we can do it!" Andrew and Ryan returned each bin to its usual place in the garage, and I praised and thanked each boy, thinking, "Wow, this is the life!" After years of tending to my *twins'* every need, my boys were now turning the tables and pitching in with our *family's* needs. As twins grow older, they can play a larger role in helping the household run smoothly. There is more to be done in your home because of the number of kids, yes, but your kids can and should learn to contribute to and help out with the numerous household tasks.

Raising twins through their early years is quite an endeavor. Parents of twins learn so much through the process, but we learn just as much about ourselves as we learn about our children. Did you know that you have an unlimited capacity for patience and love? You fed 2 babies around the clock, changed endless diapers, resolved conflicts between warring toddler twins, and so much more.

Your twin parenting skills will continue to adapt through the years as your children grow in their school years. In the early days, parents of multiples keep a synchronized schedule of feeding and constant care. Now, as your twins grow older, your job as a parent will shift to managing the psychological aspects of raising 2 loving yet independent people.

What do the school years hold in store for your family? The school years offer new challenges and choices to be made regarding academics, classroom placement, extracurricular activities, and sports. Each of your children has strengths, weaknesses, and personality quirks that will affect relationships within your family and how you parent during the school years. Over time, each child will evolve, requiring frequent reassessment to see what strategies are working and what needs to be tweaked.

Among other fun adventures coming your way is that your twins will one day be eligible for a *driver's license.* Many parents of older twins have joked with me, "It gets easier all the time, but just wait until they're driving!" We parents of multiples will navigate drivers' education and other hurdles the same way we've adjusted to our other milestones—one day at a time, one step at a time.

Now that your twins have grown past the hectic early years, the school years have their own set of challenges and issues.

## Built-in Life Lessons

Your twins learn significant life lessons simply from growing up with a sibling so close in age. They learn *patience,* as their parents have more than one child for whom to care. They learn how to *share.* They have been sharing their parents from the beginning, and as they grow, their sharing skills get lots of practice each day, as they almost always have a playmate nearby. Twins learn *empathy.* Being so close to their sibling, they develop an understanding of other people's points of view. Many experts believe that school-aged twins can be more socially savvy than their single-born peers because they have continual practice negotiating and interacting with another person.

The twin bond is beautiful and will always be special for your children and family. However, as your twins grow, continue to give your kids plenty of opportunities to be individuals and pursue their own interests. They will have different strengths, and these strengths should be celebrated. Twins will almost always have a strong relationship, but each twin will go on to make his own friends, participate in different sports and activities, and have different life experiences.

## Classroom Placement

The issue of classroom placement was initially raised in the previous chapter, specifically the Preparing for Preschool section (for more information, see pages 147–151). It is important for parents of twins to remember that the decision of classroom placement for their children is not a onetime-only decision. Every year, your children are growing and maturing, and they may have different, distinctive needs as time goes on. I strongly recommend that parents reevaluate their family dynamic each spring to determine the best path for the upcoming academic year.

**Twin Tale**

Danielle, mom to third-grade twin boys, shares, "Our twins are in different classes at school. This has always been a great balance for our family—time apart at school and time together at home. It has helped them to not compete with each other on tests and grades."

Kim, a first-grade teacher who has taught several sets of multiples, is also mom to quadruplets in kindergarten. She has special insight both personally and professionally into the issue of classroom placement for twins. She advises that it is important to identify whether your twins lean, or rely, on each other too much. Every set of twins is different. If yours are independently minded, being placed into the same classroom may not be that big of a deal.

Same-sex twins, regardless of whether they are identical or they are fraternal, may have more issues to consider regarding classroom placement compared with boy-girl fraternal twins. Boy-girl twins, by virtue of the ease with which others can tell them apart, do not have nearly the same amount of identity and independence issues that are wrapped up into the classroom placement decision. For more on this, refer to the Straight From the Source: What Twins Have to Say section on pages 188 to 191.

 **Twin Tale**

Sue, mom to third-grade twins, advises, "Be your child's advocate. Be wary of teachers who may view the children as a 'package deal,' where one child's progress is compared against the other's. They are individuals and should be treated as such."

In 2005, Minnesota was the first state to legislate that families should have the right to decide how their multiples are placed into the classroom, and since then, Illinois, Texas, Georgia, and other states have followed suit. Check to see whether your children's school has policy regarding classroom placement, and discuss your concerns with the appropriate administrative members from your district. Many districts do not have a formal written policy. In these cases, advocate on your kids' behalf. Each child's personality, needs, and learning style, as well as the twin relationship as a whole, will play a role in your decision.

Of course, twins have a special relationship, but as parents we need to be mindful of the give-and-take between siblings. If one twin tends to become shy without the comfort of his co-twin, parents should be aware and make efforts to give him increasing amounts of practice interacting with others on his own. Over the summer and during the school year, twins can participate independently in different activities or sports, which will ease the transition and help each individual be able to function to his full social and academic capacity.

 **Twin Tale**

Leigh, mom of 4, including fraternal twin girls, shares, "When our girls started school, we made the decision to keep them together. For the most part, it went very well. It was easier for me to know that they had the same homework and classwork on the same days. It helped keep me organized. They didn't seem to have many problems with having their own identity while still being in the same class. We made the decision to split them in fourth grade because they would move to a more departmentalized class schedule.... They each have their own strengths, and fortunately, we have not witnessed much sibling rivalry. They seem to be aware of what their own strengths are and seem truly happy when the other one does well. I hope this continues as they get older."

## Competition

A bit of friendly competition between twins, or siblings of any age, can be a good thing, pushing each child to her full capacity. Olympian Michael Phelps had 2 older sisters who swam, which encouraged him in his formative swimming years. Legendary National Football League quarterback Tom Brady had 3 older, athletic sisters who similarly encouraged him. Everything in moderation, though. As parents, we should ensure that the competition between our kids, multiples or not, remains of the healthy variety. And for twins, the tendency to compare is ramped up a bit. Overexuberant competition can result from twins sharing the same birthday and being in the same grade in school.

One way parents can help prevent excessive competition among their kids is to avoid labeling their kids. Your children will differ in their academic, musical, physical, and artistic talents. Be mindful, however, of whether you label your children. When a child is told she is smart or sporty, she may experience limited confidence in other areas.

Siblings, especially twins, may also subconsciously underachieve in certain areas so as to differentiate themselves from their family members. Praise your child's specific *efforts*, not the *outcome*, whether it is a report card or a basketball game. Examples include "You worked really hard on creating that poster for your class project; I like the details you included," as opposed to "You are so smart." Telling your child, "I am proud of you! You swam really hard and beat your best time," as opposed to "You came in second!" places the emphasis on effort, over which a child has more control, instead of how she placed.

From preschool through third grade, our twin boys were always in different classes. This worked really well for our family and helped each boy establish himself as an individual within their grade in school. Our boys could focus on their early education without constantly reminding teachers and young classmates who was who. Recently, my son recalled, "Back in kindergarten, a lot of kids didn't even realize I was a twin!" which, frankly, he seemed to have enjoyed perhaps because of its novelty. One day in kindergarten, as all the classes were lining up after recess, Andrew's class was instructed to line up before Ryan's. The teachers shared with me that quite a few 5- and 6-year-olds were calling *Ryan* over, telling him he had better line up, thinking he was Andrew not paying attention!

That our boys live together, sharing a bedroom, family, home, and more, means they have plenty of together time. So for us, a few hours apart during school came with the added benefit that they could appreciate each other more during after-school hours. I feel our boys get along much better with the occasional separation.

For fourth grade, we chose to have Ryan and Andrew in the same homeroom for the first time (our district rotates all fourth graders between 2 classrooms for the day's subjects). Our boys had spent the prior 6 academic years separated and for the most part did quite well with being in the same class for the first time. The novelty of it definitely was a plus.

The annual geography bee gave us a taste of competition, however. Each year, the school gives all the students in a grade the same geography examination. Each homeroom winner advances to the grade-level finals, held before all the students in the grade, and each grade-level winner goes on to compete in the school finals. Although Ryan performed extremely well on the qualifying test, Andrew was the class winner, earning the public spot of competing in front of the grade (and parents of the grade-level finalists), clearly an honor for Andrew. This made for some interesting conversations about winning and losing gracefully, and we were mindful of how we spoke with our sons, choosing our words of praise carefully. We emphasized with Ryan that it was Andrew's special time during that particular week. Other times, we would celebrate Ryan's achievements, and we would all (including Andrew) cheer for Ryan at those times.

A great strategy for a healthy family dynamic is to focus on *fairness over the long haul.* There will be some days, weeks, and even months when one child has special achievements or, conversely, particular needs or an illness. Other occasions, siblings will need more from us parents. In the long haul, it will even out. Each child will have her own day in the sun.

## Balance: Pursuing Individuality Yet Avoiding Activity Overload

Although parents know to nurture each child's interests and allow each child to pursue individual interests, including extracurricular activities, we live in the real world, with financial limits and time constraints. Especially for parents who work outside the home, simply getting multiples and siblings off to where they need to be can be overwhelming, let alone the very real issue of being able to afford the lesson fees, team costs, or other expenses. Use common sense and realize it is OK for some activities to be shared. Try not to compare your family situation with that of your neighbors' family, who may have 2 children spaced 5 years apart. Look at the big picture and prioritize those activities that are most enjoyed, eliminating less-appreciated activities when needed.

Our 4 kids were born within a 4-year span, so there has been a fair amount of overlap with their extracurricular activities. As a family, we have prioritized school as No. 1, and everything else follows. I try to follow a personal rule of school followed by religious education, a single musical instrument, and a single sport at a time to prevent an overwhelming schedule, but we maintain flexibility and do our best to honor each child's truest interests. This is in spite of today's world of year-round youth sports, which is stressful for many families. Many school-aged kids are burdened with excessive extracurricular activities, so do not feel guilty if your kids are not signed up for as much as their classmates. Unscheduled free time is just as important for their development.

Underscoring the importance of free time to play, the American Academy of Pediatrics has formally stated that free, unstructured play is a necessity for kids of all ages. When screens are turned off and kids are bored, the magic happens. Instead of adults directing the activities and determining timelines, kids who engage in open-ended play boost creativity, turn taking, and social skills and have a buffer against stress. Often these random moments are what are most fun for a child. When I was young, on rainy days my brothers and I would set up buckets and other random receptacles at the end of the house's gutter downspouts, and as they filled with rainwater, we would deliver the water to our wagon, which served as a reservoir of sorts. The grand finale of this water factory game was working together to dump the filled wagon onto the driveway. This simple activity was among my favorite childhood memories, playing with my brothers toward a silly, common goal! Look back and search your own childhood for similar memories, which will serve as inspiration for ensuring your kids have free, unstructured playtime.

## Boosting Literacy

Learning to read is a process, and the reading process begins when your babies gnaw on their first board books. Add encouragement and your kids will, over time, grow into confident readers who get absorbed into the plot of a chapter book. Research continues to show that surrounding your children with words (of both the spoken varieties and the written varieties) boosts literacy skills and nurtures a lifetime love of reading.

Each of your twins will develop reading skills at her own unique pace. Do not be surprised when one seems to take off with reading more quickly than your other. Make a dedicated effort to read to each of your twins one-on-one as often as possible, so as to work at each child's individual pace and comfort level, without her siblings interrupting the experience.

## Age-Appropriate Chores for Kids

A friend with school-aged triplets plus an older singleton shared on social media during the month of January, "It's been a successful winter break from school. Our oldest is now trained to load the laundry and measure detergent and fabric softener. [Our] triplets are trained to move laundry from washer to dryer and start the dryer. They all have to cooperate to lug

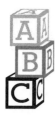

## Twin Tip

Despite having read to my children every night at bedtime and during the day, I always looked for more ways to encourage their literacy.

I found a wonderful chalkboard at our local craft store for about $2. It was simple, only measured about 7 inches by 8 inches, and was easy to stick up into a corner of the kitchen with double-sided, removable picture-hanging strips. The strips stayed together with Velcro, so I could take the chalkboard up and down every day. We started out writing kindergarten sight words on the board, but later we wrote the dinner menu on it. Our kids got a kick out of writing the menu themselves, making the board a fun way to reinforce writing skills—quite the mileage out of $2.

Message boards with removable letters and characters are also popular these days and can serve double duty as home decor and literacy boosters. Stock up (you can even put them into your kids' bedrooms) and have fun with them!

a basket of laundry up the stairs. What should the next life skill be?" We are raising future adults after all! For kids' own sakes, plus the practicality of having help around the home, parents should encourage teamwork and age-appropriate chores for *all* family members.

Kids who perform basic household tasks help the home run more smoothly, and the earlier the idea is introduced, the more it becomes the norm for a family. As kids grow, their responsibilities should gradually increase along with their skills, in a developmentally appropriate way. Early initiation of chores paves the way for preteens and teens to perform further household tasks. Contributing to the home boosts self-esteem, relieves boredom, and instills good life skills that will be infinitely useful once a teen grows into an independently living adult. In the earlier stages, resist the urge to overly help your younger child with a particular task. Yes, of course the task would be handled 3 times as fast by a parent; however, practice helps your child master the task, and kids need to start with baby steps. Applaud the effort, don't strive for perfection, and keep the big picture and goals in mind.

Always consider your child's abilities and developmental level when introducing new household tasks. For example, not all 12-year-olds have the same level of maturity and respect for safety. I include these tasks so

## Older Toddlers and Younger Preschoolers (Ages 2–3)

- Pick up toys and place into toy bins (for pre-readers, attach printed photos of what goes into which toy bin to help with sorting [eg, train bin, block bin]).
- Set table at mealtime with nonbreakable plates (eg, melamine, which is widely available) and simple flatware.
- Dust surfaces and sweep floors (recommendation: provide commercially available fiber cloths that trap dust and dirt—this can be a game for kids).
- Fetch supplies for care of younger siblings (eg, diapers, wipes, new clothes) or during meal preparation (vegetables and other simple ingredients).
- Place dirty clothes into laundry hamper.
- Help move clothes from washer to dryer.
- Make and neaten bed.
- Perform simple cleaning after arts and crafts projects.

## Older Preschoolers and Kindergarteners (Ages 4–5)

### Earlier tasks plus

- Put dirty dishes into dishwasher.
- Set table and clear table at mealtime (nonbreakable plates).
- Wipe up spills (kids should know where supplies and paper towels are kept).
- Straighten bedroom space.
- Sort clean silverware.
- Prepare a simple healthy snack.
- Dry and put away dishes.
- Use handheld vacuum to help clean messes.
- Wipe out bathroom sinks and clean bathroom counter surfaces (suggestion: use household disinfecting wipes).
- Water indoor plants.
- Feed pets.
- Fold dish towels and washcloths.
- Match clean socks.
- Clean up after arts and crafts projects, and put away supplies.

## Younger School-aged Children (Ages 6–8)

### Earlier tasks plus

- Collect trash throughout house (reuse plastic bags from stores as trash can liners for bathroom; kids can pull out filled bags and replace with fresh bags).
- Fold towels of all sizes.
- Vacuum and dust/mop floors.
- Empty dishwasher and put away clean dishes.
- Pull weeds, rake leaves, pick up sticks before lawn mowing, and sweep porch.
- Peel vegetables.
- Prepare a simple salad (wash vegetables, find ingredients, and perform simple cutting with supervision).
- Replace toilet paper rolls.
- Prepare a simple breakfast with some supervision (eg, cereal, toast).
- Wipe bathroom sinks, counters, and toilets (convenience household wipes are good for this purpose).
- Retrieve mail and newspaper.
- Wipe down microwave.
- Write needed items on a centrally located grocery list.

## Older School-aged Children (Ages 9–11)

### Earlier tasks plus

- Take garbage and recycling to curb.
- Clean toilets and clean bathrooms.
- Vacuum.
- Sweep out garage.
- Help load washer and dryer.
- Hang and fold clean clothes.
- Put groceries away.
- Water indoor and outdoor plants, including garden.
- Walk pets.
- Wipe off table.
- Prepare simple meals (eg, sandwiches).
- Help prep school lunches the night before school days.

## Middle Schoolers and Older (Ages 12+)

### Earlier tasks plus

- Clean bathroom tub and shower.
- Make full meals and plan for future meals.
- Bake cake, cookies, and bread.
- Contribute to grocery shopping list.
- Clean refrigerator and freezer.
- Mow lawn.
- Supervise younger siblings' chores.
- Change lightbulbs.
- Wash and vacuum car.
- Wash windows.
- Supervise younger siblings.

that you can plan for your child's future chores. As always, practice safety first with good instruction beforehand; make sure your child demonstrates a good handle on the tasks, good decision-making, and an understanding of how to handle situations that do not go as planned.

Mornings are a challenging time for families with twins, and many parents find it hard to get out the door on time. I'm always looking for ways to help my kids take more personal responsibility for getting themselves ready. When my twins were in the first grade, they were working on reading analog clocks and I wanted to help them apply that sense of time to their everyday lives. The twin goals of *time proficiency* and *timeliness* inspired me to post a reminder by the clock in our entryway. The project took me about 5 minutes from start to finish. I used a children's book on how to tell time that had a pretend clock with movable hands in it. I moved the hands to the appropriate positions and made 2 separate copies to illustrate the times we had needed to head out to the bus stop and when the bus would actually arrive.

If your home is anything like ours, you might find yourself repeating similar messages each day to a crowd of kids. Use your imagination to tackle some of the more common themes while boosting your kids' independence at the same time.

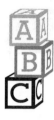

## Twin Tip

In a home filled with growing twins, you have a lot of little people eating a lot of food and a lot of little people who, over time, are fine-tuning their reading and writing skills. This tip is a simple way to boost literacy and at the same time make sure your fridge and pantry stay well stocked.

Keep pads of paper and either pencils or washable crayons in a central location of your home. Whenever any member of your family (grown-up or child) notices that you're running out of milk, bread, or even toilet paper, encourage her to write it on the shopping list. Younger kids can even draw a picture of the item or get spelling help from a grown-up or an older sibling. Practicing writing items on a shopping list is fun for kids in elementary school, and they don't realize they're gaining valuable literacy practice at the same time.

If kids are encouraged to add to the shopping list regularly, it will become a habit. You'll be instilling good responsibility, teaching each child to contribute to the household. Just don't be surprised if you walk by the list one day and see that a child has scrawled "chocolate" or another such kid-endorsed "necessity" on your shopping list.

## Teaching School-aged Twins Vital Safety Information

Even though smartphones make memorizing less necessary, your school-aged twins should learn important phone numbers. Consider maintaining a list of important phone numbers as a document on your computer, and post a printed version in a central location of your home, such as on the refrigerator. Customize your list to include any numbers you deem important. Go ahead and include your favorite takeout restaurant's number below the emergency numbers. We keep key information on ours such as

- Mom and Dad's cell and work numbers
- Grandparents' and neighbors' phone numbers
- Pediatrician office number
- School numbers and absentee hotline numbers (very handy, as my 4 kids often attended 3 different schools)
- Poison Control number
- Local pharmacy numbers, including that of the nearest 24-hour pharmacy

A paper copy of the list is always available and easy to reference, and it never needs recharging. If you head out for work, date night, or a rushed, unexpected emergency, the hard-copy list is ready for your children's caregiver with all pertinent information—no need to worry about preparing the information every time you leave the house. Just as carrying an umbrella seems to ward off the rain, being prepared for unexpected scenarios gives peace of mind. If the master document is kept on your computer, you can easily make corrections and updates as needed. Print out extra copies for nearby relatives or neighbors and they'll have your contact information ready. The list is a good example for kids to understand how to be prepared for emergencies and other various situations. Even our youngest knows where the master contact list is, and if need be, she can use the houseline to call her dad's cell phone, or Grammy, in a jiffy.

## Multiple Kids, Multiple Shoelaces

Kids master many milestones in their early years—drinking from a sippy cup, toilet training, tying shoelaces, and reading independently, to name a few. For families with twins or more, these milestones can sometimes be overwhelming, as you are teaching 2 or more children at the same age (and usually developmental level) the same new skill. The logistics of coaching 2 kids at once, while dealing with inter-twin dynamics (eg, hurt feelings when one twin catches on sooner than the other), might lead a parent to buy Velcro sneakers for life. However, once your twins achieve each milestone, their increased independence is well worth the effort.

Our strategy to teach our twins to tie shoelaces was similar to what we did for other milestones—a mix of group time and one-on-one time. Working in our favor was that our twins looked up to their older brother. We borrowed his terminology for tying shoes ("The bunny runs around a tree, jumps into the hole, and gets locked inside with a knot"). If your twins do not have older siblings, ask a beloved older cousin, family friend, or neighbor for help. A kid-to-kid demo can sometimes be more effective than merely watching a grown-up perform the task. Exciting new shoes and books about lacing shoes (with actual laces) help too. Plenty of online videos give visual, play-by-play tutorials as well. Make it fun, and know when to take a break. As your twins encounter new milestones on their developmental journey, hang in there, be patient, and treat each twin as an individual, and soon they will master the new skill of the day.

# Bedroom Spaces

If you have the ability and space to give each of your twins his own bedroom, wonderful! You can skip ahead to the next section in this chapter. For those who need their kids to share for space reasons, read on. Some families have to get creative. Jill, mom to 6, including sixth-grade twin boys, shared that recently, one boy moved out of their joint room into a tiny non-room so that he could have his own space.

Because of space constraints in our home, our twin boys need to share a bedroom. However, each boy has divergent tastes, has varying degrees of cleanliness and orderliness, and is growing and changing every day. If your twins need to share a bedroom like ours do, here are some issues to consider.

- Each child deserves protected, special space for his treasured objects and to express his distinctive personality.
- Each child needs some degree of privacy.
- Kids' interests change quite rapidly—choo-choo train decor may quickly be outdated with new interests.
- The belongings of 2 kids takes up twice the space, and the clutter can easily become a mess.

If you opt for loft or bunk beds, make sure your kids are developmentally ready for them (the American Academy of Pediatrics has safety tips at HealthyChildren.org [www.healthychildren.org/English/healthy-living/sleep/Pages/Bunk-Beds-Safety-Information-for-Parents.aspx]). Clean, simple bookshelves are a great showcase for more than a reading collection. Select 2 narrow bookshelves to conserve space, and designate one to each child to display his own treasured objects, special crafts and creations, and souvenirs from a trip, or whatever he is into that month. Furniture shopping in brick-and-mortar stores is time-consuming (and almost always an adventure with kids in tow). Instead, browse online for affordable strategies to contain the clutter, and carve out unique areas for each child.

Brainstorm together with your kids for decor that will be appropriate for longer than 1 year. I found affordable laminated world and US maps online that not only look nice on a wall but come in handy when your kids want to know the location of Peru or Transylvania.

# Family Dynamics and Behavior

Have you noticed your kids' behavior can take a turn for the worse during particularly hectic weeks? Often this phenomenon is not just a poorly timed coincidence. The overall concept of discipline is a structure in which good behavior is rewarded and reinforced, and inappropriate behavior has consequences (for more on discipline, see the previous 2 chapters, specifically the Kind and Effective Discipline section on pages 120–125 and the Consistency and Discipline section on pages 155–159). We've all heard of a time-out for poor behavior, but even more important is "time in"—positive, pleasant one-on-one time with a parent. Time in boosts your child's self-esteem and strengthens your emotional connection. Having a good relationship is wonderful in and of itself, but in addition, it is the setting under which you can most effectively guide your kids' behavior. I call it "feeding the meter." Positive quality time with a parent on a regular basis helps your child know that he does not need to act out to get your attention.

So how can you feed your kids' meters? Even if both parents work outside the home, it is possible to squeeze in meaningful one-on-one time each week. As you prep dinner, let one of your kids help with simple, age-appropriate tasks as you talk with each other, leaving the TV off. On weekends, take just one child with you on an errand, ignoring your cell phone or other distractions. Sit with your kids and simply color and doodle with them, sharing peeks at one another's artwork. Play catch with one child outside. Over time, you can fairly distribute time in among all your kids, strengthening bonds and improving overall behavior.

# Travel and Having Fun

These days, a family is considered large with more than 2 kids, so those of us parenting multiples plus singletons automatically fall into this group. Day to day, I don't consider our family of 6 particularly big because it is our personal version of normal; however, I can't help but notice the costs adding up when we buy tickets for an event or airfare.

## Budget-Friendly Outings for Twins

We often take advantage of early bird rates for a summer family membership at a nearby community pool. The school year can be hectic, so we look forward to a loosely scheduled summer break. The pool is a nice option for those pleasant lazy days when nothing in particular is on the calendar. Signing up, there is a bit of initial sticker shock (especially because many base rates are for a family of 4), but when you calculate the cost of admission for 6 family members for 2 or more visits, the numbers work out similarly. Any subsequent visits over a year's time are free. Memberships are available for your area's museums, zoos, aquariums, and more. Do the math and you might find it'll save your family some money too. Also, look for deals such as reduced–ticket price Tuesdays at movie theaters, free admission days to museums, and events at which kids younger than certain ages enter free.

Another benefit of the up-front investment of a membership is that you won't feel stressed to spend the entire day at the museum or zoo seeing every single exhibit. This membership is particularly handy when you have younger kids in your group. Too much action packed into one day can be overstimulating, and a crew with young kids will need to head home for nap time at some point. If kids are getting tired or cranky, no problem! You can leave and see the rest another time, with no additional financial cost. Many museums have reciprocal partnerships with other cities' attractions, so you can even take advantage of discounts if you're hitting the road this summer. Having a couple of family memberships on hand means not having to think too hard for activity ideas. Pack up a homemade lunch for your crew and you've got an affordable, low-stress, fun, and educational activity for the day.

## Traveling With Older Twins

With each passing year, you'll notice that outings and travel are easier and easier. This is your life, so don't be afraid to head out on an adventure, whether by car or by airplane. A positive mental outlook definitely helps. Treat the travel portion as part of the excitement, not just as a means to get to the destination. For longer car trips, prep containers ahead of time with sliced fruit and veggies, ready to go. Food prepped at home is healthier and more budget friendly than hitting fast-food restaurants while en route. Have each child pack her own backpack with books and age-appropriate activities. Visit the library or bookstore in advance so that you can pull out new books on the trip. Try to stop every 2 to 3 hours for kids to let off steam, or as I call it, get out the heebie-jeebies. Giving kids an opportunity to run around and stretch their legs helps them behave better in the car.

The American Academy of Pediatrics recommends limiting children's screen time, but on a lengthy trip, it's OK to pull out the screens for *designated* amounts of time, ideally with some kind of an educational component. Be mindful of overly long stretches of screen time, as your kids will become zombielike, and a lot of kids can get motion sickness if they don't regain their sense of balance and horizon by simply looking out the window from time to time. Our family uses a timer on road trips, with designated chunks of time, aside from screen time, for conversation, car games, and snacks.

For air travel, it may be worth the investment to purchase each of your multiples a small, wheeled bag in which to carry a beloved teddy and activities onto the flight. Families with twins need more stuff, so put your kids to work by having them help carry the load in an age-appropriate way. Your younger travelers will enjoy feeling like a jet-setter, pulling their own wheeled mini-suitcase! When possible, choose direct flights to reduce traveling mayhem and disruptions.

## Adolescent Multiples

Someone wise once told me that by the time your child reaches 12 years of age, she already knows your parental opinions on pretty much every subject under the sun. The teen years are a time to modify our interactions with our kids, making sure we are present for our kids, ready to listen. Listening to your children as they develop independence is a great way to let them know you trust them to think for themselves.

Communication is key. Often the best conversations occur when the pressure of a particular topic is offset by the environment in which the conversation is held. For example, talking while driving is a great way to connect. Somehow, when both parties are looking forward toward a destination, a bit of pressure is released, and teens are often more likely to offer information. Similarly, chatting while putting away laundry or performing other household tasks together, such as washing dishes after dinner, is a great way to reconnect and catch up on various subjects. My favorite way to connect with my son Ryan, even after 15 years, is playing catch in our yard. We are silly—he loves for me to throw the ball randomly to challenge him to make a difficult catch (I'm sure our neighbors think I have zero ball-throwing skills as a result!), but then we also can catch up (pun intended) on what's going on in our lives. Also, a big step toward good family communication is ensuring that screen time is monitored. Make sure screens are put away during mealtimes and at least an hour before bedtime.

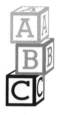

**Twin Tip**

Great books to read when your multiples are tweens or teens include *Building Resilience in Children and Teens: Giving Kids Roots and Wings,* 3rd Edition, by Kenneth Ginsburg, MD, MS Ed, FAAP, with Martha Jablow; *How To Raise an Adult: Break Free of the Overparent-ing Trap and Prepare Your Kid for Success* by Julie Lythcott-Haims; and for parents of girls, *Untangled: Guiding Teenage Girls Through the Seven Transitions into Adulthood* by Lisa Damour, PhD.

If your tween or teen shares a particular dilemma or issue with you, resist the temptation to jump in immediately with suggestions on how to handle the situation. Allow the conversation to breathe, as this gives some space for your teen to come up with potential ideas and solutions herself. This involves asking questions such as "What do you think about that?" to prompt further introspection. After years of helping our kids, it can be a bit of a role shift to intentionally step back and encourage self-reliance and resilience, but it is important to do so. Besides giving teens increased practice making decisions for themselves, it also sends an important message that you trust and respect their opinions and ideas, which boosts self-esteem. The importance of strong self-esteem in adolescence cannot be overstated, as it can ward off unhealthy relationships with peers and unhealthy risk-taking behaviors.

## Straight From the Source: What Twins Have to Say

When my boys were in kindergarten, we played the board game Candy Land. When one of them landed on the same space as his twin, he exclaimed, "Look, we're *double* twins!" When they were in first grade, some-one asked Ryan, "What does it feel like being a twin?" He shrugged and responded, "Pretty normal." Around that same time, I tried to explain to them what it was like when I was pregnant with them. Two babies squeezed into one belly (for several months, no less) is quite a concept. My boys began telling jokes about how they spent that time together, and through endless giggles, they agreed, "We were playing checkers!"

**Twin Tale**

Here are some other goofy questions my identical twin sons have heard.
- **Do you ever mistake yourself for your brother?**
- **Do you ever think you're Andrew? (directed to Ryan)**
- **I know people ask you this all the time, but who are you? (Ryan and Andrew note that both adults and kids have asked them this.)**

Here are what some other twins have to say about their experiences.

Jill, who grew up with a fraternal twin brother, is now a mom to sixth-grade fraternal twin boys herself. Her experiences growing up as part of a boy-girl twin team give her special insights into parenting her twin boys. She shares, "Their main sport is basketball, and they have always made the same team. However, this past fall, they both played a different sport. They *loved* having it as their own."

Dani, an identical twin and mom to 3 girls, including twins, shares, "My first-grade teacher suggested we switch classes to fool [my sister] Kara's teacher. The teacher didn't guess! It was only when I took my shoes off and the teacher told me to put them back on that another student told her, 'That's Dani, not Kara.' After that, we switched one day every year and the students always could tell, but the teachers [couldn't]. Another time, we went to my grandparents wearing customized shirts with our names on them, only switched. When we told them that we were really the other twin, they didn't believe us! Now that we're adults and she lives overseas, most people in my life don't even know I'm a twin."

Alexis, along with her twin brother, are juniors in high school. She shares, "We appreciate how our parents look at us as individual people and not as a unit. We were encouraged to seek out our own interests (hobbies, sports, music, etcetera) and are not compared in our accomplishments. This may have been easier for our parents, as compared to some parents of twins, since we are different genders."

Madeline and Catherine are identical twin girls in fifth grade. They share, "We have a special bond with each other that is hard to describe but is stronger than our bond to our other sisters and our friends."

Brian, now a dad to twins himself, grew up with an identical twin brother. He says, "In general, it bothered me when people would ask, 'Are you the good one or the bad one?' Really, people, who asks kids that question? And no, if you punch him in the leg, I do not feel his pain!"

Shelby and Payton are 8-year-old twin girls. Shelby says, "You always have someone to stick up for you if someone is bullying you." Payton says, "The best thing about having a twin sister is you always have someone to have your back." Their mom, Michelle, shares, "I love that they watch out for one another without smothering each other."

Taylor and Jaden are 8-year-old twins. When asked what they want others to know about being a twin, Taylor said, "It is hard to share the same birthday." Jaden wanted classmates and family members to know "We are not identical."

Emily and Jack are 9-year-old twins. Jack shares, "It's hard when one twin is doing better than the other in school or sports. But it is good to have a built-in friend because if you are bored, you can ask [her] to do something." Emily shares, "Twins can be different, especially boys and girls. It's OK to do different things—sports, interests. I wish my friends knew that twin brothers aren't annoying. Sometimes it's not fun to have to play boy games, but I do it because I know my brother doesn't like to be alone."

Emily and Maddie, 10-year-old fraternal twin girls, share, "Sometimes it is hard to be a twin because you have to share everything and people get you confused. It is [also] fun because you always have a person to play with and talk to, and you always have someone to support you and stick up for you." Their mom, Leigh, mom to 4 kids total, adds, "Our twins are like night and day, and it is hard to see people expecting them to have the same disposition and personality. I am thankful for the unique personalities they...have."

Lois, 90 years old, grew up with an identical twin sister. She comments on the generational differences for multiples, between her youth and these days, now that multiples are more commonplace. "My mother always dressed us alike. We were 'special,' as there were not many twins in our hometown—really, anywhere. We always loved the attention that we got from the public, from complete strangers who would always comment that we were twins. We recognized our own strengths and weaknesses. We were our own best friends; we had each other and were the 2 youngest of 5 girls. We did the typical swap dates, who happened to be our future husbands. They didn't even know they were with the wrong twin. We only told them when they put their arms around us. We all laughed because they had no idea. Another time, I was asked out on a date, but the young man actually wanted to ask my twin. He just didn't know who he was asking out. We were always in the same classes; everyone got confused without us actually doing anything. We loved going to [Twinsburg], Ohio, and seeing hundreds upon hundreds of twins!"

# CHAPTER 9

# Support, Emotional Health, and Time-savers

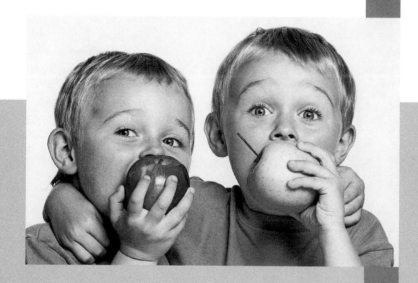

My childhood friend Lisa parents boy-girl toddler twins and 3 older siblings, and it has been a joy to follow the adventures of her growing family. I marvel at how her family and each of the families I know who have twins or more have parenting journeys that are uniquely theirs. Well-meaning friends and family offer you advice, which is wonderful. Yet sometimes with this advice, you often hear a variation of "Been there, done that." Nope! No one has walked in your shoes, no one has had your specific family structure, and no one has parented your unique children. Every family's situation is distinctive and different.

When her twins were first born, Lisa received advice on how to best raise her babies by anyone and everyone. Sometimes the advice was solicited and sometimes not. Taking a walk in public with a hugely pregnant belly is the best way to attract attention and comments from random strangers passing by. When I visited Lisa after her delivery in the hospital, her nurse came in to check vital signs and told her, "You know you *have* to feed the babies 30 minutes apart, right?" Lisa, aware that I am a big fan of feeding baby twins simultaneously, smiled and said, "OK, thanks!"

Here's the deal: although others may have parented children, although others may have raised twins or triplets, *their experience is not your experience.* Listen to the advice and well-wishes of others, but find your own path. Some twins are born first to a family. Some triplets are born third, fourth, and fifth to a family with 2 older kids. Some of us have local family members able and willing to help, while others do not. Each family's needs are different, and each situation or circumstance affects how you handle baby feeding schedules, bedtime routines, naps, and more. Your neighbor's method for soothing her infant's colic may not work for your infant. Some babies love swings; others, not so much. You only know once you try it out.

|||||||||||||||||||||||||||||||||||||||||||||||||||||||||||||||||||||||||||||||||||||||||||||||||||||||||||||||||||

## Parenting Tip

Borrowing unnecessary baby equipment is a great idea. When our twins were babies, we borrowed a swing that was still in a good and safe condition—thank goodness because none of our 4 kids were a fan of it. We didn't waste any money on an item that would have sat in the corner taking up space.

|||||||||||||||||||||||||||||||||||||||||||||||||||||||||||||||||||||||||||||||||||||||||||||||||||||||||||||||||||

When offered advice from others, smile gratefully and store it in your mental notebook. Give it a try if it sounds reasonable, and feel free to tinker and experiment to see whether their strategies work for you. But remember that you know your children better than anyone on this planet. Once you've ensured your children's health and safety, sometimes a certain degree of flexibility, with a dash of trial and error, is needed before determining how to best tackle the current parenting stage or challenge.

New parents of multiples need all the support, tips, and encouragement possible, and while no single book fits all families, parents need support and troubleshooting tactics to handle the myriad issues involved with raising multiples. Each family creates its own rule book, and no two will look the same. I aim to *empower* parents of multiples like you to gather information and advice, use common sense, speak with your pediatrician, and see what works best for *your* family.

## The Teamwork of Raising Multiples

When you have 2 or more newborns to care for, both parents need to roll up their sleeves and get to work. Some fathers may not have planned on being a hands-on type of dad, yet when twins are born, more manpower is needed. Out of necessity, very quickly these dads become proficient in feeding, burping, and changing diapers. Such tasks are necessary and significant opportunities to connect with your children. Feeding and diaper changes are ideal times for parent-child communication and bonding. Hands-on fathers not only have more fun, compared with noninvolved parents, but also boost their children's development by providing a different kind of interaction from that experience with the other parent. As an example, Mom may be gentle and nurturing, while Dad may be goofy and blow more raspberries on their babies' bellies. The combination of 2 different styles leads to a more well-rounded experience for your children.

### Parenting Tip

To use a basketball analogy, parents of singleton babies play 2-on-1 defense, parents of twins play man-to-man defense, and parents of triplets or more play zone defense, my personal favorite. The teamwork involved in parenting twins benefits both your kids and your partnership.

# Seeking Support

Reach out to extended family and friends during your pregnancy to establish "help lines" to assist with the challenges lying ahead. If possible, designate one close family member or friend to act as a contact person who organizes help with tasks that must continue despite possible bed rest and the birth of multiples (eg, preparing meals, housecleaning). Online resources are available to coordinate a meal chain for a family blessed with multiples. Meal Train (www.mealtrain.com), CareCalendar (www.carecalendar.org), and Take Them a Meal (https://takethemameal.com) are some examples of websites dedicated to organizing assistance with meals and ensuring that multiple meals aren't delivered on a single day.

## Parenting Support

Amber, mom to 4 kids, including fifth-grade identical twin girls, recommends, "Have a support system in place to help you; you will need it. If someone offers help, take it! Multiples are overwhelming, and it's OK to have those feelings that maybe this is not going well. I was already a mother, so I thought, 'How hard can it be?' Well, a lot harder than I thought. The best advice I would tell my 32-year-old self is don't be so hard on yourself; you really are doing the very best you can. Those babies are doing just fine."

If finances allow, a sitter, "family helper," nanny, or designated night nurse can help ease the chaos of the early weeks with multiples. Examine your budget, if necessary, to tighten elsewhere to make it possible to hire help. Our family was fortunate to have the help of a local middle school student who was eager for more experience with kids. Her help progressed to full-fledged sitting, and she came over often as a family helper to play with our older children when our fourth child was born. A great bond was formed, and as the years progressed, she has been a significant person in our children's lives. When she was a college student, she was a fabulous summer sitter for us when home on break.

## Parenting Tip

Meal planning, both by prepping meals and by freezing meals ahead of time, can help immensely once your babies are born.

Child Care Aware is a useful resource for families looking for quality child care close to home. For more information on nannies, au pairs, and home-based child care providers, please refer to the Early Infancy and Getting on a Schedule chapter, specifically the Returning to Work section on pages 74 to 75.

## Parenting Tale

Jon, dad to infant twins, says, "Though by no means a simple or haphazard personal expense, hiring a night nurse for a majority of the nights in a week to take over feeding, changing, etcetera, has been an invaluable decision, worth every penny. We 'tag teamed' the night feedings and care with our first singleton and managed to come out fine, albeit a bit exhausted, on the other side. With [our] twins, if we didn't have a night nurse and instead were doing everything ourselves, neither of us can conceive just how unproductive the rest of our lives would [be]."

Families expecting multiples should reach out for local support through their communities and places of worship. More specific to families with twins, triplets, and more, multiples organizations (on the local level as well as state and national levels) support families through both in-person meetings and online social networking groups.

### Necessary Household Tasks

Whether you're put onto bed rest pre-delivery, trying to survive the first couple months post-birth, or you're parenting school-aged multiples, running a household can be quite challenging. It can be helpful to make a list of all the necessary household tasks. Once you determine all the necessaries, you can strategize and decide which tasks are a priority for you, what should be picked up by your partner, and what should be delegated to loved ones or outsourced financially. Check your budget for room to make help possible. Tasks to consider include
- Cleaning
- Grocery shopping
- Meal planning
- Assistance during bath time and bedtime
- Lawn service
- Repair or maintenance work

## Multiples of America

The Multiples of America organization serves to support families raising multiples, to advocate for education and research in the field, and to foster friendship and community. Their website, www.multiplesofamerica.org, has a search function to help you find a Parents of Multiples club in your area, either by zip code or by city.

Parents of Multiples clubs usually hold monthly meetings that provide camaraderie and support. Often each monthly meeting has a guest speaker on or topic related to raising multiples or parenting in general. Clubs often hold separate, more casual gatherings to get the kids together or to arrange for a mothers- or fathers-only outing. The Parents of Multiples club that I was assigned to during my twin pregnancy held monthly meetings on a night of the week that my husband regularly worked late hours, making it difficult for me to attend some meetings. Fortunately, I lived in the populated Chicago suburbs, and I was able to investigate alternative local options, which included a smaller, cozier club that met a different night of the week and was a better fit for me, personality-wise. Don't be afraid to investigate different options to better fit your needs.

Seasonal clothing resales are often held twice a year and are a fabulous way of not only finding excellent deals on baby clothes, equipment, and toys but also passing them along when your babies have outgrown certain items. Parenting 4-month-old twins does not leave one with much free time. Add in other kids, work, maintaining a household, and finding time to eat, sleep, and exercise properly, and not much time remains to maintain friendships, let alone seek new ones. Yet maintaining those social lifelines, as well as making new connections with other parents of infant multiples, can be rejuvenating.

### Parenting Support

When our twins were younger, I was doubtful that I had the time to attend my local Parents of Multiples club monthly meetings, yet when I was able to swing it, I was so grateful I did. There is something instantly comforting about sitting in a room full of people who *get it*. Sharing tricks, tips, and ideas (and sometimes venting) about the twin parenting experience can be downright soothing for your soul.

Social media platforms allow families with multiples to connect online with local and regional multiples groups as well. Several groups are public (watch for the globe icon, which indicates anyone can read the posts, photos, and comments), but many groups have a private forum to post questions and suggestions, making it even easier to stay connected, even if you are unable to leave the house for a meeting. If you belong to public social media groups, be mindful that your posts and photos may be viewable to anyone. Keeping your kids' privacy in mind when navigating social media is important.

|||||||||||||||||||||||||||||||||||||||||||||||||||||||||||||||||||||||||||||||||||||||||||||||||||||||||||||||||||||

## Parenting Tip

Michelle, mom to third-grade twin boys, shares, "The single most important advice for me when I was pregnant with my twins was to get into a support group or some kind of monthly activity that [gives] you time away from the kids. When you get a chance to step away, even when there is so much to do, it gives your mind a rest and you feel refreshed."

|||||||||||||||||||||||||||||||||||||||||||||||||||||||||||||||||||||||||||||||||||||||||||||||||||||||||||||||||||||

## Emotional Support

A study published in the April 2009 issue of *Pediatrics* struck a personal chord with me. The article "Multiple Births Are a Risk Factor for Postpartum Maternal Depressive Symptoms" states, "Undergoing a high-risk pregnancy and delivering multiple births are stressful life events, and the unique demands of parenting multiple infants can result in high levels of parental stress, fatigue, and social isolation." Looking back at my twins' early months, housebound by the needs of twin babies plus a 1-year-old, I agree with this statement.

The study results, though not surprising, are vital. With this study, families and health care professionals can anticipate and understand the relationship between multiple births and stress. Knowing that the odds of depression are greater, families can enter the world of multiples with their eyes open, ready to be proactive with some prevention strategies.

In the early months with twins or triplets, prioritize what is most important and streamline elsewhere. You cannot do it all. Ask yourself whether each of your kids is safe, fed, and loved. If yes, declare the day a success—the other stuff can slide for now.

Some parents' outlook may improve with day-to-day logistical help or talking with loved ones, but others may need counseling and further assistance to get on the right track. If you are feeling overwhelmed, you are not alone. Be a squeaky wheel, and reach out for support.

Be *specific* in how you ask for support. Instead of vaguely hinting, ask your partner *directly* for what you need. For example, "Please change the babies' diapers." Necessary tasks that may seem apparent to you may not be clear to others. Don't expect your partner to read your mind.

Good communication between parents is key, as is tapping your wider support circle. Friends lend an ear so that you can vent, and relatives with older kids remind you that your kids' current stage will soon pass. The parents in your local Parents of Multiples club truly understand what you're going through. Also, look to your place of worship and to your pediatrician, who wants to know how *you* are faring. Your babies' growth and development are intricately related to your family dynamic.

||||||||||||||||||||||||||||||||||||||||||||||||||||||||||||||||||||||||||||||||||||||||||||||||||||||||||||||||||

### Parenting Tip

Darwin, dad to school-aged twins, recalls that as the parent working outside the home each day, he knew that he would come home to a house in which things had to be taken care of, and he would need to help out. Their babies did not always stay on routine, so patience was needed.

||||||||||||||||||||||||||||||||||||||||||||||||||||||||||||||||||||||||||||||||||||||||||||||||||||||||||||||||||

## Mental Health: Keeping the Big Picture in Mind

Georges Seurat's *A Sunday on La Grande Jatte* is one of the better-known works of art in the Art Institute of Chicago collection. It was featured in the movie *Ferris Bueller's Day Off* and was the inspiration for Stephen Sondheim's *Sunday in the Park with George*. Seurat used the painting technique called *pointillism*. Looking at the canvas up close, you can see individual dots of color, but from a distance, the big picture, a scene of people enjoying a park, unfolds.

I mention painting techniques to illustrate a mental health point. When faced with parenting challenges, we often find ourselves standing too close to the canvas, unable to see the big picture. Every child is different, and our initial strategies to help our kids navigate developmental milestones may be hitting a brick wall. If we remember to step back and observe the scene as a whole, we can refresh our perspective. By reestablishing our priorities and goals and rebooting our parenting energies, we'll be able to see the forest for the trees.

How do we reboot? Parents need to take personal breaks to maintain sanity and nurture ourselves. Parents should ensure that they have an outlet, an activity, or a hobby unrelated to parenthood or their careers that nourishes the inner spirit and rejuvenates them for engaging and caring for children. This is challenging during your multiples' early weeks, but especially after your babies are 6 or so months of age, it is something to think about.

Look at a typical week's schedule and see where your personal protected time can be squeezed in. Even the busiest of us can use creativity to unearth 30 minutes, 3 times a week, for this purpose. Enlist the help of your partner, family, friends, or sitters to make it happen. Also, consider waking up earlier than your family (if not too limiting on your overall sleep), or when your babies are older and have more consistent schedules, use the magical time between their bedtime and your bedtime.

Meeting our own needs helps us properly care for others. My husband and I work together to cover for each other, protecting each other's time weekly. Whether you exercise; are an avid photographer, scrapbooker, or gardener; or love to experiment in the kitchen with new recipes, make an effort to set aside time each week to pursue your passions. Your family will be rewarded with a refreshed parent who has the big picture in mind. On the most challenging days? At the end of the day, ask yourself, "Is everyone safe and fed properly?" Then declare the day a success!

## Keeping Your Cool

Keeping a cool head when your children misbehave is challenging. Handling 2 or more young kids at the same age can test the patience of a saint. It is crucial for parents to stay calm in the heat of a discipline moment for many reasons, because kids learn how to handle stressful situations by observing how their parents handle such situations.

One tip to preserve your emotional health as a parent, especially when your twins are toddlers and your patience is being tested daily, is to review the developmental milestones and characteristics of your kids' age-groups. HealthyChildren.org is a great resource to remind yourself of appropriate stages. Families can find some comfort knowing that it is *age appropriate* for older babies, toddlers, and even preschoolers to test limits. Unfortunately, toddlers' tantrums are also age appropriate. They result when your 2-year-old realizes she has her own ideas about the world and realizes she is, in fact, a separate person from her parents and her twin. (For more on toddler discipline, please see the Toddler Years [1- and 2-Year-Olds] chapter, specifically the Kind and Effective Discipline section on pages 120–125.)

Throughout your twins' early years, they are continually trying to figure out what their boundaries are. This process is a function of how children operate and is *not* a conscious, deliberate attempt to drive you crazy. As frustrating as the tough days can be, it is our job as parents to consistently and rationally illustrate appropriate boundaries to our kids. For an excellent resource on your children's progressing developmental stages, refer to the American Academy of Pediatrics *Caring for Your Baby and Young Child: Birth to Age 5.*

How can you model reasoned, rational behavior to your kids when you have reached your capacity for patience? Counting to 10 and going to your "happy place" may not be enough to keep you, a parent of multiples, calm. Some goofy yet effective ideas to stay cool include imagining an audience in the room with you (or security cameras, or the camera crew from a reality TV show) watching you as you handle a tough situation. Alternatively, you can pretend your toddlers are from another country and you're teaching them the ways of your land. Silly ideas, but sometimes, tricks are just what parents need to remain calm and handle a situation objectively, properly, and without anger.

## The Built-in Benefits of Multiples

While we raise our twin sons, I keep adding to an ongoing, lengthening list of the benefits of parenting more than one child at the same age.

- *Self-reliance.* Kids learn self-reliance early on when they outnumber their parent(s). Believe it or not, being outnumbered can be a good thing. The very logistics that pose such a challenge in the first year after birth encourage your children to become more independent as they grow and develop over time. We've all heard of helicopter parents who can be overly involved in their kids' lives and activities. Parenting twins or more decreases the chances that you'll be micromanaging each aspect of your kids' experiences. I have a personal tendency to swoop in and help too much; however, with 4 kids born within 4 years of age, I can help each child only as much as humanly able. By the time they were school-aged, my kids were pros at preparing their backpacks for school, packing school lunches, helping put away laundry, setting the dinner table, and more, not necessarily because of my parenting skills but because of the logistics and needs of our larger-than-average family.

- *"You can't scare me; I have twins!"* Once you've parented multiples for any stretch of time, you realize you are capable of more than you may have expected. You quickly learn the ropes and can handle a multitude of situations, which is empowering. This sense of empowerment can carry over to other areas of your life, such as handling your career and your personal relationships. If you've raised multiples through the exciting first year, you can handle anything.

- *Resilience.* Multiples coach their parents on how to roll with things and adapt. Time flies quickly when parenting multiples; we tackle current issues and then move on to a new set of circumstances. Even during a difficult stage, rest assured: time will pass, the stage will pass, and you'll be onto the next milestone.

## Healthy Family Dynamics

Do you sometimes worry that your twins get too much attention, leaving their younger sibling on the sidelines? Or are you like a friend of mine who worries that her toddler twin boys are neglected because of their older sister's busy schedule of school and activities?

When 2 or more children are involved, well-intentioned parents do their best to maintain a fair family dynamic by providing equal amounts of love and attention to each of their kids. These efforts can be fraught with guilt, however, as it is *impossible* to provide exactly equal amounts of interaction with 3, 4, or more children. Life is just so variable—how *could* your attention be spread equally? One week, kid No. 1 is sick. Another week, kid No. 2 has a school play. Then the following month, kid No. 3's best friend moves out of state. I often find myself fretting if I have not had enough special time with one of my 4 kids, even if there are very good reasons that some kids needed more of me during any given week.

Having twins or triplets in a family can intensify the issue of relationships. By their very nature, multiples are a rare, special occurrence, and they are fascinating as well as time-consuming. I have friends who happened to grow up as a single-born sibling of twins. They warned me, when I was pregnant with my twins, to not forget my oldest son. These warnings intensify my feelings of guilt during those hectic weeks when some of my kids get more attention than my others.

I think the best strategy for a healthy family dynamic (and fret-free parents) is to focus on *fairness over the long haul*. Some days, weeks, and even months, one of your kids will need you more than your other(s). And that is *OK*. Over the long haul, it will all even out, and each child will have his own special moments with you and your partner.

## Time-saving Strategies

Time is a tricky thing. We have 24 hours each day to spend as best we can. Families with multiples need to use time-saving strategies whenever possible. Manipulate your daily schedule to budget your time effectively. Creative thinking can streamline your home's daily tasks and make your life easier.

Take dinner prep, for example. When your twins are newborns, the dinner hour is the bewitching hour. New babies tend to become more anxious and unsettled during the late afternoon and early evening hours, and colicky episodes usually peak right at dinnertime. What superhero could cook and serve a meal while also caring for 2 fussy babies? Even as your twins grow into toddlers and preschoolers, they may be bouncing off the walls come late afternoon. During their school years, your twins are getting off the bus in the afternoon and have homework and various extracurricular activities scheduled. Frozen pizza 7 nights a week isn't the healthiest option, but the forces of the universe seem aligned in a mission to thwart homemade dinners forevermore.

The solution? Prepare dinner in advance at a time convenient for you and your schedule, and then assemble or reheat it right at mealtime. I am a morning person and my kids, when little, were usually more agreeable and cooperative in the morning hours. If able, I would assemble lasagna, to be baked later, or roast chicken parts so that they would require only a microwave reheating. A slow cooker is a valuable kitchen device for this strategy, with countless online recipes. Come 5:00 pm, most of the prep is complete, and even if it is a hectic afternoon, you can quickly toss together a decent meal for your hungry family. Mornings aren't the only alternative. Families with busy work schedules may find that weekends are a good time to assemble a few nights' meals in advance. Alternatively, pressure cookers are now popular and make healthy meals in a fraction of typical cooking times. See what works for your family and your situation.

---

## Parenting Tip

If you need to make a trip to the grocery store and don't have time to make a list, take a picture (or several) of the inside of your refrigerator with your smartphone to see what things you have or don't have and the amount that is left.

---

You can twist time to make it work for you. Dinner can be made in the morning. Laundry can be done when your kids are in bed. Prime time TV shows can be watched on demand for relaxation, if that is your scene. Hectic mornings can be alleviated by placing backpacks into the car the night before. Identify your trouble spots and experiment with new strategies, and you'll find yourself a more relaxed, and more effective, parent.

## Strategies for Special Occasions

Holidays and birthdays are terrific occasions to get together with family and friends. However, when you have young babies, your day-to-day life can be hectic enough. The thought of hosting a get-together can be daunting. Consider the possibility of making your life easier by hosting at your home, as opposed to traveling a distance to visit a family member's home for the holiday. Think about it. Your twins' cribs, all your baby supplies, your milk, and even your changing table are at home. Having your loved ones come to your home means that you don't have to pack and travel.

Most important, your children will be happier and healthier if they consistently have a routine nap and nighttime sleep schedule, even on holidays and special occasions. From time to time, life will inevitably get in the way of a perfect schedule for your kids, but if you can entertain at your home on a holiday, it will be easier to respect your kids' normal routine. Striking a balance between routines and flexibility will serve your family well in the long run.

An easy way to host a gathering is to plan for side dishes and desserts that can be made a day ahead of time. Then on the day of the event, all you need to do is focus on a main dish and reheat the rest as needed. This plan not only frees up your event day but also spreads out the cleanup of prep dishes over a few days' time. Better yet, delegate the sides, beverages, and extras to your guests to bring as potluck items. It is not cheating to get a little help from the grocery store either. Hummus is an example of an appetizer that you can open up and scoop into your own dishware to make it your own, if that makes you feel better. It will taste great, and you as the hostess will be happy and relaxed, not overworked and exhausted from adding more prep bowls to the dirty dishes.

Family get-togethers are about loved ones gathering, not about how clean the house is or what food was served. I'd recommend prioritizing and not fretting about a perfectly clean house before the event. Often the gathering is so fun and boisterous that no one is analyzing the cleanliness of your home. If they are, too bad for them! Keep this as your focus and you'll be a calm host, ready to enjoy your own holiday.

---

### Parenting Support

Michelle, mom to 8-year-old twin girls and a 13-year-old singleton, states, "My girls make me laugh every day. They have taught me so many things like to appreciate the little things in life. A spotless house isn't as important as the tea party they are having. Even though days are sometimes hard and seem like they are never going to end, when a little [one] takes your hand and asks to go snuggle and read stories in the 'big bed,' everything else can wait for a moment. Cherish those moments. Important lesson learned. Whether outside on a sunny day or dancing in the rain, imagination is a wonderful thing. I find it's important to be silly with them."

---

## Modified Expectations

I once read a holiday "survival" article in our local newspaper. It had good advice, yet I believe that the year-end season is not a hardship to endure; rather, it is a gift. Parenting twins or more keeps you busy *every* month of the year. During this month, as with any month, prioritize what is truly important and enjoy the spirit of the season without overwhelming your-self or your children. Despite various family, social, and religious events, *you* are in control of your schedule for the most part.

Embrace your most treasured traditions, such as an afternoon spent decorating cookies with your kids or taking your family to see glorious outdoor light displays. Make time for these experiences by saying no to items lower on your priority list. You can't do it all. Realistic expectations for the holidays, especially when your twins are young, can help maintain some serenity. Traditions from years past can be reevaluated as well.

Saying no may be difficult for many of us, but we often need a reminder that we have permission to do so. We owe it to ourselves and to our children. Your infant twins cannot speak up for themselves, so you need to be their proactive advocate. If you avoid overscheduling, you'll prevent meltdowns, illnesses, and behavioral setbacks. I am not endorsing the life of a hermit who declines all outside invitations; rather, I am suggesting *balance* in how you spend your precious family time. This may be a difficult concept for grandparents to understand, especially if your multiples are the first grandchildren on one or both sides of your family. They may have preconceived notions of you visiting, and that may or may not be feasible. I encourage you to remember that as a parent, *you* are now in charge of your own family, and you have the authority to make these decisions for yourself and your children.

Ultimately, keep in mind that your twins' early years are fleeting. Accommodating the needs of young twins is a temporary situation that will be just a blip on the radar screen over the course of your lives. Streamline your days during holiday months to enjoy each member of your family, your traditions, and the true peaceful spirit of the season.

## Finding Lessons in the Mishaps

Years ago, when my kids were small, during a particularly hectic week for our family, I decided to take it easy and pop a frozen pizza into the oven for dinner. The timer rang and the pizza somehow broke into 2 pieces upon removal, resulting in big glops of cheese, sauce, and bell peppers falling onto the oven floor and racks—so much for a painless dinner.

Was I happy about the now-smoking oven? Definitely not! However, my usual audience of 4 little kids was watching to see how I would handle this unexpected suppertime dilemma. I decided to laugh about it and call my kids over to watch (from a safe viewing distance) as I attempted to extricate some of the burning cheese blobs. At the time, my kids were 7, 5, 5, and

3, so of course they found this entire scenario hilarious. We then rallied together to open as many windows as possible, laughing at the mess Mom made, hoping the smoke alarms didn't start blaring.

How do children learn to deal with mistakes, disappointment, and difficult situations? During early childhood, parents and other important caregivers model attitudes and coping strategies, whether they are aware of it or not. Keeping this in mind, I consciously chose to take the lighthearted path and joke about the smoking oven.

Despite our best efforts, we parents are human and our kids will see us lose our cool from time to time. Do not fret if that occasionally happens; emotions are a part of life. If you've found yourself yelling or otherwise exhibiting less-than-model behavior, it is OK to simply talk with your kids about it (eg, explaining that you shouldn't have used those particular words). Use daily life events and mishaps as illustrative scenarios to help your young children learn to navigate their emotions and maintain their self-esteem, even when things go wrong. It's healthy for kids to see that we all have good days and not-so-great days. You're raising future adults, who need to know how to move forward from the inconvenient bumps in the road.

## Where's the Answer Key?

Do you ever wish there were right and wrong answers to your parenting dilemmas? A nice, clear-cut, straightforward way to go? It sure would make life easier! As your children grow and your family's dynamics evolve, parenting quandaries will arise that have no obvious correct answer.

When our then 5-year-old twins were ready for new bikes, we had a dilemma of modest proportions. We had a perfectly good hand-me-down bike, courtesy of our older (singleton) son. So who would get the hand-me-down bike, and who would get a new bike?

Our solution: I tossed a coin to determine who got the new bike, and we figured that in a couple more years, when our boys needed bigger bikes again, we'd alternate between our twins as to who got the hand-me-down and who got the new. My son who lost the coin toss was pretty bummed, and I started to feel pangs of guilt as I reassured him. Nothing that I said, though, made him as happy as when he simply hopped onto and rode his bigger and faster bike, beaming with pride at how much he had grown! A bonus was that he had instant gratification; his hand-me-down was ready to go, waiting in the garage for him. His twin who won the coin toss had to wait for his new bike to be assembled from the box.

There may not be an exact answer key for your parenting dilemmas, but remember that regardless of the paths you choose, kids are resilient. Each family and each child is unique, so follow your instincts with love and fairness, and you'll make the right decision for *your* family.

# CHAPTER 10

# Preterm Birth and Other Birthing Challenges

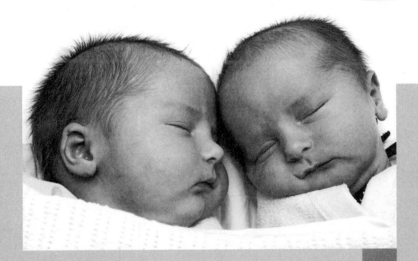

ost twins do well after delivery. However, multiples have a greater chance of preterm delivery compared with single-born babies. This is a sensitive subject and is not meant to scare you; rather, this chapter provides an overview of issues that preterm babies might face as well as some terms and therapies that a family may encounter in the neonatal intensive care unit (NICU), should they find themselves in this situation. If you are pregnant with multiples, do your best to keep a positive spirit and healthy outlook on your pregnancy, but familiarize yourself with some of the following issues to prepare in case your family experiences preterm delivery. Any challenge is better handled with preparation ahead of time.

According to the American College of Obstetricians and Gynecologists, *preterm birth* refers to all deliveries that occur at fewer than 37 weeks of gestation; this classification includes

- *Very preterm* (less than 32 0/7 weeks)
- *Moderately preterm* (32 0/7–33 6/7 weeks)
- *Late preterm* (34 0/7–36 6/7 weeks)

The fractions in these gestation time periods range from 0/7 to 6/7 and indicate additional days per a 7-day week, because every day in the womb counts. *Term birth* refers to deliveries that occur from 37 0/7 to 42 0/7 weeks, and *post-term birth* refers to any delivery occurring after 42 0/7 weeks.

Newborns born between 34 weeks of gestation and 36 weeks of gestation (near, or late, preterm births) make up most of all preterm births in the United States, and in 2007, the American Academy of Pediatrics recommended a change in terminology from *near term* to *late preterm* to better describe the special health concerns of newborns born at these dates.

A term pregnancy is 37 weeks or longer, yet twin babies usually deliver, on average, around 36 weeks. The National Vital Statistics Reports (NVSR) from the Centers for Disease Control and Prevention (CDC) showed that 60% of twins born in 2016 arrived before 37 weeks of gestation. The final weeks of pregnancy are a time for your growing babies' weight gain and lung maturation. For this reason, if your babies are born early, they may face low birth weight and respiratory difficulties.

The 2016 CDC NVSR statistics further illustrate that 20% of twins were born "early preterm," meaning at fewer than 34 weeks of gestation, increasing the chances of the therapies and treatments described in this chapter.

Triplets were born before 37 weeks of gestation 98% of the time in 2016, with 66% born before 34 weeks. Quadruplets were born before 37 weeks 97% of the time, with 93% born before 34 weeks.

Some multiples who are born a little early may need time in the NICU to gain weight before going home. Other babies may have respiratory difficulties in addition to needing to gain weight. More significantly preterm twins may have additional issues. Each newborn is evaluated and treated individually, and it is possible that each newborn may have dissimilar needs at birth. Preterm deliveries can be scary for parents and families, but the good news is that modern medicine has made wonderful advancements in the care of preterm babies.

Being born preterm does not necessarily mean lifelong health issues. Wayde van Niekerk set a new world record for the 400-meter event at the 2016 Rio Olympic summer games, winning a gold medal. He was born at 29 weeks' gestation and weighed 1 kilogram (2 pounds 3 ounces) at birth! Also, the Litherland triplets, successful competitive swimmers, one of whom has competed at the Olympic level, were born preterm. Their parents involved them in swimming at an early age for the specific purpose of helping develop their lungs (see the A Glimpse Into the Twin Experience chapter, specifically the Multiples and the Wide World of Sports section on pages 253–255). Mission accomplished!

||||||||||||||||||||||||||||||||||||||||||||||||||||||||||||||||||||||||||||||||||||||||||||||||||||||||||||||||||||||||||

### Parenting Tip

For more valuable information about newborn intensive care, an excellent resource is *Understanding the NICU: What Parents of Preemies and Other Hospitalized Newborns Need to Know* edited by Jeanette Zaichkin, RN, MN, NNP-BC; Gary Weiner, MD, FAAP; and Davia L. Loren, MD, FAAP, from the American Academy of Pediatrics.

||||||||||||||||||||||||||||||||||||||||||||||||||||||||||||||||||||||||||||||||||||||||||||||||||||||||||||||||||||||||||

# The NICU: Different Levels of Care at Different Hospitals

The NICU is a special place that most people, including parents, might not be familiar with, unless they have family or loved ones who have already required the services of a NICU. Most families who are expecting single-born children don't necessarily include familiarity with the NICU as part of their planning and pregnancy preparations; however, because multiples tend to deliver early, it is wise to be aware of what the NICU is all about.

## Parenting Tale

Kim, mom to quadruplets, recalls, "When I was on bed rest in the hospital, they gave us a tour of the NICU [neonatal intensive care unit] facilities ahead of time. This was very helpful. I saw that the NICU had an open area, in which all the babies were cared for; there were no private rooms. They showed us a baby who was about the size that they expected my babies to be when born; that was a surprise. Usually, when you see pictures of babies, they are larger full-term babies, not the reality of what a premature baby looks like. Although even with this advance preparation, the NICU experience is totally different when it is your own children being cared for."

Talk with your obstetric team about your delivery hospital options. Be aware of the different levels of care available at different hospitals. If your pregnancy has been monitored by a maternal-fetal medicine (high-risk) team, you will likely have more information about the level of care available for your babies after delivery. Every hospital can handle emergencies, but many community hospitals prefer to transport pregnant women at higher risk to the region's medical center, where staff is more experienced at managing complicated pregnancies and sick newborns.

In 1976, the March of Dimes categorized obstetric and newborn and infant services at hospitals as Level I, II, or III, depending on the availability of resources and the complexity of patients served.

Here is a breakdown of each of these levels.

- **Level I:** Basic nursery services, designed to care for healthy term babies. Babies born at fewer than 35 weeks of gestation are transferred to another facility.
- **Level II:** Nursery services designed to care for babies born at more than 32 weeks of gestation who weigh more than 1.5 kilograms (3 pounds 5 ounces). This level of nursery has been further divided into Level IIA and Level IIB, with Level IIB having the capacity to care for babies who need mechanical ventilation (ventilator) or continuous positive airway pressure (also known as CPAP), a form of support for babies with breathing problems, for a day or less.

- **Level III:** A subspecialty service that offers comprehensive care for all newborns. Often located in a regional medical center, this type of facility is equipped to provide neonatal intensive care. Level IIIA cares for newborns born at more than 28 weeks of gestation who weigh more than 1 kilogram (about 2 pounds 3 ounces), while Level IIIB cares for newborns born at fewer than 28 weeks of gestation who weigh less than 1 kilogram. The Level IIIC NICU provides the highest category of care for the most complex issues, including those that require extracorporeal membrane oxygenation, or ECMO, which is cardiac or lung bypass, and complex birth defects that require surgical repair.

Early in your pregnancy, talk with your obstetrician about how your pregnancy is progressing and what will be the best facility with the proper resources for your babies.

||||||||||||||||||||||||||||||||||||||||||||||||||||||||||||||||||||||||||||||||||||||||||||||||||||||||||

### Parenting Tip

Kristine, mom to first-grade triplets, shares, "All the staff and nurses in the NICU [neonatal intensive care unit] were awesome. The only scary part was seeing my babies with all the wires, breathing tubes, etcetera. But the nurses were so great at explaining everything, so that gave me comfort."

||||||||||||||||||||||||||||||||||||||||||||||||||||||||||||||||||||||||||||||||||||||||||||||||||||||||||

# Nutrition

If you are physically able, you can start pumping breast milk soon after delivery. Breast milk is the perfect nutrition for small or preterm babies. Pumping your milk regularly helps boost your milk supply. If your babies cannot yet tolerate feeding by mouth or a nasogastric tube (often called an *NG tube*), which goes from the nose to the stomach, the milk can be frozen and fed at a later date. A high-quality, hospital-grade breast pump can help you double-pump breast milk quickly and easily. Recruit your nurses and the hospital lactation consultants for assistance and advice. Your neonatologist (newborn pediatric specialist) may recommend boosting the calorie content of your breast milk with human milk fortifier (also known as HMF, a powder that increases the caloric and nutritional value to the milk, such as adding iron).

Breast milk is ideal, but there are also formulas specially made for babies born before 36 weeks. Several options have more calories per ounce than standard formulas to maximize your newborn's or infant's nutritional and energy requirements, a key step toward growth and proper catch-up weight gain. In addition, supplemental iron will help boost preterm babies' blood supply.

Your preterm baby may not yet have developed the suck and swallow reflexes. Babies who cannot yet suck and swallow from a bottle may benefit from nasogastric tube feedings, during which breast milk or formula is fed via a small tube that enters through the nose and leads to the stomach. Tube feeding helps the stomach and intestines stay healthy and accustomed to digesting milk until the baby develops her own suck reflex.

## Parenting Tale

Kim is mom to first-grade quadruplets born at 29½ weeks and recalls her family's neonatal intensive care unit (NICU) experience: "The hard part was the ups and downs. You would have what seemed like a good day with progress made only to get a call at one in the morning with a problem that one baby was experiencing. To describe the NICU, you go through a journey where you take one step forward and 2 steps back. Then 2 steps forward, 2 back, and so on until you are moving forward without regressing. It seems like an eternity to get there, but you do. Developing a strong relationship with the NICU nurses is hard and emotional but also critical."

# Conditions Commonly Treated in the NICU

## Respiratory Difficulties

During the final weeks in the womb, the lungs form a substance called *surfactant,* which helps the lungs develop elasticity, like a balloon, to open up and take air more easily after delivery. Babies born early may lack this substance and may develop respiratory distress syndrome (RDS) as a result. Corticosteroids such as betamethasone are usually given to a mother in preterm labor before 34 weeks to help prevent RDS. If a baby has signs of severe RDS, surfactant treatment is given to the baby soon after delivery and in the first couple of days after birth, and the baby will require the help of a breathing tube and ventilator. Babies with less severe RDS may require a nasal tube with oxygen. Preterm babies who require supplemental oxygen for longer periods may go on to develop chronic lung disease (CLD).

Chronic lung disease is not the same thing as chronic obstructive pulmonary disease, or COPD, which affects adults. For babies born early, CLD, also known as bronchopulmonary dysplasia, or BPD, refers to persistent inflammation, injury, and scarring of lung tissue that occurs because of underdevelopment of preterm lungs and the treatments needed to support the immature lungs. It's not possible to predict what a baby's life will be like on the basis of what occurred during the NICU stay. In other words, even kids who require intubation and ventilation for any amount of time may do better than expected. At the time of this writing, I am mentoring a medical student in my office practice who was born in the 1980s at 26 weeks' gestation. She's an intelligent and fantastic young woman well on her way to becoming a physician herself!

The longer a baby is on a ventilator, the more likely that preventive medications will likely be needed when the baby is discharged home from the NICU. The length of time can be quite variable, and it depends on the child and his progress. Some children require daily preventive medications (possibly including inhaled medications with a nebulizer machine) for the next couple of years, while others may require medications only during the winter months of cold and flu season. And still others may do quite well on their own without specific prescriptions. Babies with respiratory concerns should be monitored closely by their general pediatrician and a pediatric pulmonologist for at least a year after going home from the NICU.

Preterm babies commonly have apnea of prematurity, which means they have episodes when they forget to breathe, requiring stimulation to continue breathing. Stimulant medication can help control apnea of prematurity, which usually resolves by the time the baby is at 40 weeks of post-conceptional age.

## Parenting Support

Reach out to other families who have had neonatal intensive care unit (NICU) experiences with their children. Sue, mom to third-grade twins, shares, "I had just found out I was pregnant when a close friend delivered 28-week[-old] twin boys. I honestly had never seen a breast pump before, let alone a premature baby or a NICU. I was very fortunate to have my friend as a resource during my pregnancy and the immediate weeks following my twins' birth. My twins were born at 32 weeks, with a 4-week stay in the NICU. Her advice to me during that time was invaluable."

## Jaundice

Jaundice is a yellowing of newborns' skin and eyes. It happens when a chemical called *bilirubin* builds up in the new baby's blood. Bilirubin is a by-product of old red blood cells and is removed by the liver. Most newborns, even if healthy and term, have some degree of increased bilirubin level because the immature red blood cells of a newborn break down more quickly. In addition, the liver is immature and not fully handling the extra bilirubin.

A simple laboratory test measures the amount of bilirubin in the blood to evaluate the degree of jaundice. Pediatricians are concerned about jaundice because high levels of bilirubin, if left untreated, can cause deafness or brain damage. Light phototherapy can reduce the bilirubin levels if needed. A baby receiving phototherapy looks like a baby visiting a tanning salon. Skin exposure helps the treatment be more effective, and the baby will even wear mini-sunglasses to protect his eyes.

---

### Parenting Support

Amy, mom to preschool-aged twin boys who were born at 24 weeks, shares, "The only way to keep moving every day is to think *when,* not *if.* When will your baby be off the ventilator? When can you hold him? When can you bring [him] home?"

---

## Other Concerns

- Low-birth-weight or preterm babies who need help maintaining their body temperature are placed into radiant warmer beds or incubators.
- Infections are a concern for preterm babies with an immature immune system.
- Babies born extremely early will require eye examinations to screen for retinal problems, as well as head ultrasounds to evaluate for any bleeding from fragile blood vessels.
- Some babies have patent ductus arteriosus (PDA), when a normal fetal connection within the major heart vessels does not close after delivery the way it should. A PDA can be treated with medication. If the medication fails to close the connection, surgery may be required.

# Bonding in the NICU

Give your babies names as soon as possible. Naming your babies will help your family and hospital staff bond with your babies. Get to know the NICU staff. They are knowledgeable and will become part of your extended family. Bring in family photos and special mementos for each of your babies' bedsides.

Initially, it may not be safe for parents to hold a preterm baby. When your babies are medically stabilized, you will be able to hold them and participate in direct skin-to-skin contact with them, which is great for *both* parents and is as beneficial for parents as it is for babies. Parent-child bonding thrives on the sense of touch.

## Parenting Tale

Kristine, mom to first-grade triplets, shares, "One regret I have is not going to the NICU [neonatal intensive care unit] often. As long as you are a patient in the hospital, you can go anytime you want, as long as the NICU team is not doing their rounds. One of the nurses called me once at 2:00 am to see if I wanted to come see Rocco. I was thinking to myself, I wish I had known, and I would have been there every night. At the time, they had 3 nurseries—NICU, intermediate, and the regular nursery. Everyone was in the NICU, and Isabella and Ava left after a day, but Rocco stayed for 3. I did have a lot of nurseries to visit, but I could have had extra visits with Rocco in the wee hours."

As your babies grow in the NICU, you will be able to become more involved in their day-to-day care. You'll learn when your babies' care times are, and you can help take temperatures, change diapers, reposition your babies, and even give baths. Continue pumping breast milk and breastfeed your babies one at a time if you are able.

# Going Home

One of your babies may be able to come home before your other. Babies who are ready to go home from the hospital should be able to regulate their body temperature, be able to take all their feedings by mouth, be gaining weight in a steady pattern, and have a home plan for any ongoing medical issues.

Your babies may need breathing and heart rate monitoring at home. Hospital staff will train you to learn how to use any necessary equipment. If one baby is able to come home before your other, use the opportunity to get into a routine before your other baby comes home. When both babies are home, coordinate feedings and nap times to occur at the same times each day.

---

### Parenting Support

Kim, mom to quadruplets born at 29½ weeks, shares, "I was so used to reading monitors in the NICU [neonatal intensive care unit] to know how my babies were doing that when I got home and there was no monitor, I was so scared that there would be a breathing problem and I wouldn't know. When my first baby came home, I think I woke her up 4 times throughout the night to make sure she was still breathing."

---

If your babies were born before 35 weeks of gestation, needed oxygen at birth, or are still on oxygen, ask your pediatrician about monthly injections to prevent respiratory syncytial virus (RSV). In older kids or adults, RSV manifests similarly to a bad cold, but unfortunately, babies born preterm or who have CLD can develop a serious lung infection if they catch RSV. In addition, ask your NICU staff and your pediatrician about developmental clinic follow-up appointments to monitor your babies' developmental growth after being discharged from the hospital.

## From the NICU to Beyond

Your multiples may have quite different medical needs whether born very preterm, moderately preterm, or late preterm. Good communication continues to be important as you work with your team of physicians and therapists. Your general pediatrician should serve as your children's medical home, helping coordinate specialists and necessary developmental, speech, and other therapies. Continue to write down concerns and questions as they occur to you during the course of a busy week so that you can ask the appropriate people at a scheduled office visit or during an additional phone call. Believe in yourself and your abilities as a parent to advocate for your children.

# Facing Infertility

If your parenting journey included fertility issues, you are not alone. The road to parenthood may have been circuitous and taken more time than your family expected, perhaps years. Acknowledge your wide range of emotions if this is the case. If your path included miscarriage, take the time and support necessary to begin to process this. Once you are able to bring your babies home, loved ones may expect you to be happy and somehow healed, yet your emotions may still be conflicted. It is important to care for yourself if you are to care for others. Seek support and mental health resources if need be.

## Double Love: My Journey to Parenting Multiples

*Andrea Z. Ali-Panzarella, DO, MPH, FAAP, FACO, Pediatrician and Child Abuse Pediatrician*

I never even thought about the possibility of facing infertility.

My journey began in January 2012, when I had my first miscarriage, an ectopic pregnancy, for no known reason. Although I am a pediatrician, it took me a long time to remember that infertility is a medical diagnosis. It is not something that my husband and I had to face; it [is] a condition that we were both diagnosed with. I quickly gained a greater understanding of what my patients endure. It has been 7 years and counting, and our journey is not over. The number of tests were too numerous to count. I had multiple surgeries and in vitro fertilization (IVF) procedures. My body has seen years of medications, along with side effects, that it would have never seen otherwise.

Falling into the statistical population of the least likely scenario, I was left with many questions unanswered. The despair, sadness, depression, anger, confusion, desperation, hurt, and anxiety seeped into spaces of emptiness when I was not looking. My silence about it all was deafening. Although I was very aware of the importance of my mental health, something had to give and take a back seat when I only had so much time and energy. However, years of multiple failed IVF attempts and miscarriages, along with unexplained infertility, lead to the recommendation of having a gestational carrier, someone who would carry our biological babies for us. This was the best decision I ever made, because I now have beautiful twin boys, and the hardest thing I have ever done, because I had to be apart from them for 9 months.

Infertility affects every aspect of your life—marriage, family relationships, friendships, work, hobbies, vacations, and social outings, to name a few. Many find it difficult to comfort those they know experiencing infertility and

## Double Love: My Journey to Parenting Multiples (*continued*)

miscarriage. This leads to even more isolation and loneliness. Losing a baby is devastating, something no one should have to experience. Your world is turned upside down and inside out. You may never really learn skills to cope with death effectively, especially when it comes to miscarriage.

I remained in survival mode until the boys' first birthday. Now, I cannot stress enough the importance of finding professional support for your mental health. As my wise therapist told me, pregnancy is not the cure for infertility. Parenthood is not the cure for infertility. Many people have tried to normalize the experience by thinking we should be happy now. Unfortunately, our current journey is not all joy. My husband and I will always have to face the emotions that come up, oftentimes unexpectedly, and we continue to honor our angel babies we lost along the way.

There are feelings about being a new parent, a parent of twins, and a parent who is on the other side of infertility. It can be confusing, conflicting, and filled with guilt. The silence continues because talking about anything negative comes with fear that someone will judge you. I allow myself to feel all of it, knowing that nothing will ever impact how grateful I am every moment of every day. This has made parenting twins even more enjoyable.

The thought of going out in public with twin babies was overwhelming and anxiety provoking. For me, conversations about pregnancy, questions about twins in the family, and comments about the finality of my family planning are very difficult to navigate. My first experience was bringing home 4-day-old twin newborns on a plane. Even going to the store was challenging. I never knew what stranger would make an innocent comment, and I was not prepared to respond. Do I tell this person my story? Do I just play along and pretend? Is this lying? Am I not honoring my babies if I don't speak my truth? In the end, though, the decision I make with each encounter ends up being the right one for my family.

Today, I have a new perspective on parenthood and what it really means to have our boys here with us. Every single day I am in awe of the miracle that it is to have twins. The level of appreciation and love that my husband and I have for them cannot be expressed in words. They will never be "double trouble"; they will always be double love. This is our family story.

I have found my voice in my boys and I am now breaking my silence. My hope is to help others break their silence and know they are not alone in raising their babies after infertility.

# CHAPTER 11

# Triplets, Quadruplets, and More

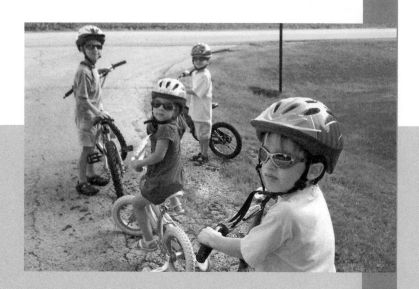

Our twin boys are 18 months younger than our oldest son, so when our family goes out and about, even after all these years, strangers and passersby often ask us whether our sons are triplets. Even though we had 4 kids within 4 years, our kids were born on 3 different birthdays, which is a much different scenario than if we had triplets plus one, or quadruplets. I have an incredible amount of respect and admiration for families with multiples, given the unique challenges they face in the early years. All families with multiples can benefit from the lessons families with triplets or more have learned to streamline care for their infants and keep their family organized.

I have spoken with many wonderful families with triplets or quadruplets, and all of them have different family structures and family schedules. Some have both parents who work full-time, some have one parent who stays at home to care for their children, and others have a parent who is back at school to further his education. Despite dissimilar family structures, these families' successes have some consistent themes, such as *organization* and *teamwork*.

## Pregnancy Preparation

Parents of triplets or more need to be prepared for a preterm delivery. Please refer to the triplets and more statistics on preterm delivery in the previous chapter, on pages 213 to 214. Mothers carrying triplets or more should expect to go on some form of bed rest around the 20-week point of the pregnancy. The bed rest may take place at home initially with modified activities and then advance to fully hospitalized bed rest. Mothers of triplets need to eat considerably more calories daily to help their babies grow. Some moms find protein shakes are a healthy and convenient way to obtain extra calories.

Even during the pregnancy stages, parents of multiples can join local Parents of Multiples clubs as well as internet support groups (for more on this, please refer to the Support, Emotional Health, and Time-savers chapter, specifically the Multiples of America section on pages 199–200). Reaching out to other families with triplets can provide practical survival tips and reduce feelings of isolation. Triplets and higher-order multiples are rare occurrences in the population, and connecting with others is emotionally helpful. Many social media groups and pages specifically deal with various stages of triplets' lives, from pregnancy through the teen years.

While you are pregnant with your multiples, begin to research various options to recruit volunteers to assist your family during the challenging early months. Ask family, friends, neighbors, and your place of worship for support. It would be helpful to designate a point person (a close family member or friend) to coordinate such tasks as a meal-train plan to which others can contribute. You will be immediately busy with the pregnancy and delivery of your babies, so assigning this task to a third party may prove useful and stress reducing.

## Synchronized Schedules

Most triplet families stay sane the first exciting year after their babies' birth by coordinating their babies' feeding and nap schedules. Families that start out feeding their babies on a more casual on-demand basis quickly find themselves overwhelmed and then need to adjust to streamline the process.

Often when babies are sent home from the neonatal intensive care unit (NICU), they will already have a consistent NICU feeding schedule, such as every 2 or 3 hours. Many triplet families take advantage of the existing NICU schedule and keep their babies on the same pattern upon their homecoming, tweaking their 3 babies' schedules to work together more efficiently. (For more on the NICU experience, please refer to the previous chapter.)

In the early weeks and months, many families obtain help with the frequent feedings. With a second adult's assistance, baby triplets can feed at the same time. One adult can feed 2 babies simultaneously, while a second adult feeds the third. If a parent handles the 3 babies solo, 2 babies are fed simultaneously followed by the third. Breastfeeding moms can breastfeed 2 of their babies together and then feed their third baby a bottle of pumped breast milk.

### Parenting Tale

Take advice from Kim, mom to kindergarten-aged quadruplets and a first-grade teacher herself. She incorporated her professional skills into methods that managed the first year with quadruplets. "We had stations for all the major tasks—a food station to prepare the milk and bottles, a diaper station, a bath station, and so on."

# Surviving the Early Months

Different families have different strategies for handling the challenging weeks when they first bring their triplets home. Volunteers can help immensely during the daytime and nighttime. Ask your helpers to perform specific duties. They can feed your babies, do laundry, cook or bring along a meal, clean the house, or just hold your babies.

Many families arrange to have help with the first month of overnight feedings. One family that I spoke with had help from relatives. Their grandmother arrived at the home each evening to handle overnight feedings for the first month their triplets were home. She would leave in the morning to refresh and return again the following evening.

Some families have their babies sleep in the same room initially and split their babies up later as needed, usually into boy or girl bedrooms for multisex triplets.

## Parenting Tip

Stash important supplies (eg, diapers, burp cloths) in convenient places on each level of the home to minimize time spent running around retrieving necessary items. Along these lines, if you find yourself repeating certain tasks daily, brainstorm ways to streamline the process and keep items related to that task close at hand.

Friends can help families organize meal programs. One family's church arranged a schedule to deliver meals to the house 3 times a week in the early months. Families find it beneficial to give helpers and volunteers very specific instructions of what needs to be done to minimize confusion (eg, how much to feed each baby, how often to pause for burping breaks, how long to hold their babies upright after feeding). Don't be shy with how you ask for assistance and what assistance you ask for. This is not the time to be proud and try to do too much yourself. Especially during the fall and winter months, make sure all volunteers are healthy, are virus-free, and receive their annual fall flu vaccine to protect your babies.

## Organizing the Multiples Way

Organizing bottles, nipples, and formula streamlines the feeding process. Many families buy supplies in bulk and store them in a designated location, to quickly assess what supplies are needed before embarking on another shopping trip.

Dry-erase boards are very useful for families with multiples. Many use a dry-erase calendar to keep track of volunteers in the early months at home. Other families use large dry-erase boards to keep track of their triplets' feedings, wet and dirty diapers, moods, and medications. As your triplets grow older, the dry-erase boards can transition to keep track of school calendars, assignments, and extracurricular schedules.

### Parenting Tip

One family with school-aged triplets and 3 older, single-born children created a buddy system in case of emergencies such as a house fire. Each older sibling was instructed to take his or her assigned baby and exit the house quickly if need be.

A mother of older triplets uses her smartphone to help stay organized. She programs in her children's appointments, school functions, and activities, and she has the phone beep 24 hours ahead of time as reminders to keep her on schedule.

Color-coding helps families with multiples keep track of each child's items. Give each child a signature color starting in infancy to help identify personal items and identify who each child is in pictures.

## Toilet Training

Families with multiples often find toilet training 3 or more kids at once to be overwhelming for everyone involved. One family began toilet training their triplets at the same time, but as their mom describes it, "It was a circus!" They abandoned that idea and began training each child separately, starting with their child who showed the most signs of readiness, with much greater success. The extra one-on-one attention each child received with separate training led to better successes on the potty. (For more on toilet training, please refer to the Toddler Years [1- and 2-Year-Olds] chapter, specifically the Toilet Training section on pages 127–132.)

## Parenting Tale

Kim, mom to kindergartener quadruplets, shares, "Toilet training was one of our more difficult stages. Each child ultimately had to decide when [he or she was] ready. One of our girls trained first, which inspired 2 of her siblings. We used incentive charts to keep everyone motivated. Further along, however, our daughter who was the first to train did have a few months of regression, and [she] needed a few more months to get back on track."

# Interpersonal Relationships, Individuality, and Emotions

How can partners support each other during the early challenging months? Sleep deprivation affects everybody's mood and can affect even the strongest of partnerships. Many families find that a consistent, early bedtime for their children gives parents some quality quiet time together. Other families squeeze in good adult conversations whenever possible—even if at 3:00 am, if that is the only time that both parents are awake and together—with no disruptions.

When navigating the early years with triplets, a go-with-the-flow attitude helps. Once one stage or schedule is mastered, things change (yet again) and you need to adapt. Try to anticipate and be prepared for your triplets' next developmental stage.

Be realistic in what you can accomplish in one day. Lower your daily expectations if you must! The early months can be a haze of constant feeding and care; take things one day at a time. A calm parent is a more effective parent.

Try not to stress about the need to give each of your triplets identical experiences. Strive to be fair among your children instead. One mother of triplets noticed that one of her triplets hit his milestones a bit earlier than his siblings and was a bit more self-sufficient. It is now years later, yet she still feels twinges of guilt about him. She worries that he missed out on some of the motherly attention that his siblings received for being needier. You cannot give your children identical experiences. You've just got to do your best to be fair, not equal.

Most families notice that as their triplets grow older, each child exhibits unique talents. One family I know had a son who excelled at baseball. They encouraged him and noticed that his self-esteem blossomed, while his siblings participated in completely different activities. It is wise not to place all your kids into a single activity. Rather, encourage each child to find his special area of interest.

Triplets can be quite a team. They are socially savvy because they are almost always interacting with other children their own age. They always have one another, and they tend to be quite outgoing in new social situations. Being raised as a triplet or more provides plenty of built-in life lessons. Triplets have learned to share and be patient from infancy, by virtue of their family logistics, and have a less self-centered view of the world because they have siblings the same age.

The importance of treating all your children as individuals, regardless of birthdays, cannot be overstated. One triplet family I know has a terrific method of ensuring quality one-on-one time with each of their children weekly. On Saturday mornings, Mom has a special outing with one child, Dad has an outing with another child, and their remaining children stay at home with a trusted sitter. A rotating schedule is used to be fair to everyone and help their children know what to expect and when their special time is coming. Even in a large family, with a bit of planning and strategizing, families can spend quality one-on-one time with each of their children.

## The Adventure of a Lifetime

Families with multiples agree that the early weeks and months are challenging, but they are more than worth it. Organization and streamlining strategies help families with triplets or more stay sane and happy. Enjoy each of your child's stages. As the expression goes, "The days are long, but the years are short." Very quickly, the stage will be over and you will all move on to the next chapter!

# CHAPTER 12

# Multiples:
# Facts, Lore, and More

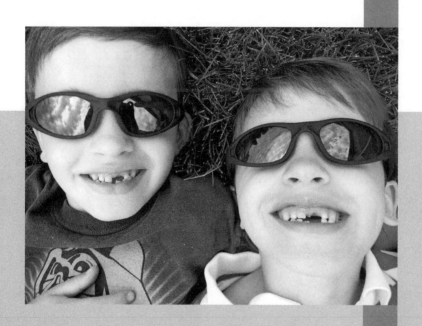

*D*o twins run in your family?" "Are they identical or fraternal?" Parents of multiples are no stranger to such questions. Just try to run a quick errand, kids in tow, without people stopping you to inquire about your family history. It's time to dispel some myths and separate fact from fiction. Now that you are a parent of multiples, your multiples' community is relying on *you* to help spread the truth!

Twins can be either identical or fraternal. *Identical* (monozygotic) twins result from a single fertilized egg that has divided into two, giving each twin identical genetic material. *Fraternal* (dizygotic) twins result from 2 separate eggs being fertilized by 2 separate sperm, giving each twin different genetic material.

Identical twins represent about 1% of all births around the world. Identical twinning seems to be unrelated to family history, maternal age, or ethnic, geographic, or socioeconomic patterns, and it has so far eluded explanation as to its occurrence. So even though everyone will still ask whether twins run in your family, and even though there are plenty of instances when an individual who is a twin herself may conceive identical twins, statistically, identical twins do not run in families.

Fraternal twins, on the other hand, can and *do* run in families. Fraternal twins have varying percentages of occurrence in different populations and places in the world. Fraternal twins are associated with a family history of twinning, advanced maternal age, and the use of fertility treatments. A family history of twins affects the maternal lineage, meaning that the tendency to produce twins is carried only by the mother, not the father. A twinning family history is a tendency of mothers to ovulate more than one egg at a time in a single monthly cycle. Despite the popular belief, twins do not skip a generation because these ovulatory events (ie, how many eggs mature in a single monthly cycle) are random each month.

Triplets, quadruplets, and more may have different variations of genetic material. For example, all 3 babies may be genetic siblings (ie, fraternal, or all developed from 3 separate fertilized eggs), or there may be interesting combinations. A pregnancy may begin as 2 separate fertilized eggs (meaning fraternal twins); however, one zygote may further split into two, meaning that the babies will be 2 identical twins plus a fraternal triplet.

# The Distinction Between Identical Twins and Fraternal Twins

Because fraternal twins are 2 separate fertilized eggs, they develop 2 separate amniotic sacs, placentas, and supporting structures. Identical, or monozygotic, twins may or may not share the same amniotic sac, depending on how early the single fertilized egg divides into two.

If twins are a boy and a girl, they are obviously fraternal twins, as they do not have the same DNA. A boy has XY chromosomes and a girl has XX chromosomes. Girl-boy twins occur when one X egg is fertilized with one X sperm and one Y sperm fertilizes the other X egg.

Sometimes, health care professionals identify same-sex twins as fraternal or identical by ultrasound findings or by examining the membranes at the time of delivery. The best way to determine whether twins are identical or fraternal is by examining each child's DNA. Occasionally, a family is told that their twins are fraternal because of placenta findings when they are in fact identical. Other times, a family may see the minor differences in identical twins and declare their twins fraternal because of these differences in appearance.

A few commercial laboratories, for a fee, will send DNA collection kits to families to help determine whether their twins are identical or fraternal. The families swab the insides of each child's cheek for a DNA sample and send the kit back to the laboratory to await results.

We were initially told our sons were fraternal twins because they had 2 separate placentas and supporting structures. However, because of natural curiosity, a concern for future medical issues, and the fact that our boys had countless physical similarities, we decided to use a commercial DNA kit to determine their zygosity once and for all. (I had initially planned to wait until our boys were at an age that they would understand and learn the news themselves with us; however, I was too impatient to wait!) The kit was easy to use, and we had our results back in a quick turnaround time. Our suspicions were confirmed, and our boys are identical—very handy if one of them ever needs a replacement kidney down the line and our other would like to help!

Identical twins have the same DNA; however, they may not look exactly identical to each other because of environmental factors such as womb position and life experiences after being born. Our family jokes that one of our twins received stitches for a lacerated upper lip because he wanted to distinguish himself from his identical twin brother. In addition to being affected by life's bumps, bruises, and differing hairstyles, a child's DNA is constantly adapting from that child's experiences. Different stretches of one's DNA can turn on or off in response to environmental surroundings; therefore, over time, a pair of identical twins' DNA becomes more and more distinctive. Whether fraternal or identical, all twins are truly 2 separate, unique individuals.

# More and More Multiples: The Statistics

If you feel like there are more multiples these days compared with when you were a kid, you're not mistaken. Multiples (twins, triplets, and more) are more common these days than a generation ago.

## Statistical Trends of Multiples

The National Vital Statistics Reports showed that the most important trends leading to the rise in multiple births are maternal age and the use of fertility treatments. Older women, without any intervention, have a higher chance of ovulating 2 eggs during a single monthly cycle. In addition, women who undergo fertility treatments or hormone therapy to induce ovulation are more likely to ovulate multiple eggs. The recent decline in triplet and higher-order multiple birth rates has been associated with updated guidelines from the American Society for Reproductive Medicine and improvements in assisted reproductive technologies such as in vitro fertilization (IVF). That is, fewer embryos are transferred per IVF cycle. In 2009, 19% of all twin births and 34% of all triplet and higher-order births were estimated to have been conceived with IVF.

Where do the most twin births occur in the United States? Multiple birth occurrence ranges widely by state. Interestingly, the National Center for Health Statistics report showed that for the years 2009 to 2011, twins accounted for 2.5% of births in New Mexico, compared with 4.5% in New Jersey. Twin rates were greater than 4% in Connecticut, Massachusetts, and New Jersey for this 3-year period. State-specific triplet and higher-order multiples ranged from 0.06% in Montana to 0.2% in New Jersey; 3 states reported triplet and higher-order birth rates higher than 0.2%: Nebraska, New Jersey, and North Dakota.

On average, most single-baby pregnancies last for 39 weeks. Pregnancies with twins average 35 weeks; for triplets, 32 weeks; and for quadruplets,

29 weeks. For more on pregnancy, please refer to the Preparing for Your Twins' Arrival chapter on pages 11 to 30.

---

### Multiples Birth Rates

Each year, the Centers for Disease Control and Prevention National Vital Statistics System publishes reports analyzing birth data along a wide variety of characteristics. The rate of twin births rose 76% from 1980 to 2009, but the pace of increase has slowed in recent years. From 1980 to 2004, increases averaged nearly 3% a year, but from 2005 to 2011, the pace of increases slowed to 0.5% each year. In 2016, the twin birth rate was 3.3% (33.4 per 1,000 total births per year), essentially stable for the years 2009 to 2012.

The higher-order (triplets and more) multiple birth rate was also essentially unchanged from 2010, at 101 per 100,000 for 2016 (roughly 0.1%), and is at the lowest level reported in the past 2 decades and down 29% since 1998. The decline in more recent years is a change from the rapid increase from 1980 to 1998, more than 400%. In 2016, triplet and higher-order births included 3,755 triplets, 217 quadruplets, and 31 quintuplets and higher-order multiple births.

---

## Twin Lore and Twins Around the World

Stargazers know that Gemini, Latin for "the twins," is a well-known constellation in the starry night sky. Castor and Pollux were twin brothers who were transformed into the constellation, according to Greek and Roman mythology.

The Yoruba tribe in Nigeria has the highest dizygotic twinning rate in the world (4.4% of all maternities). Some attribute the high twin rate to a diet high in yams; however, because the tribe clearly has a strong family history of fraternal twins, this plays a large role in the continued trend.

Each summer, Twinsburg, OH, is host to the Twins Days Festival, the country's largest gathering of multiples, with several events over the course of a 3-day weekend. You can learn more about the Twins Days Festival at https://twinsdays.org.

## Guinness World Records and Multiples

The Guinness World Records state that the most prolific mother ever achieved her status with the efficiency of giving birth to multiples on several occasions. The wife of Feodor Vassilyev (1707–1782), a peasant from Shuya, Russia, had a total of 69 children. With 27 pregnancies in all, she gave birth to 16 pairs of twins, 7 sets of triplets, and 4 sets of quadruplets. Numerous sources support this story, suggesting that while improbable and statistically unlikely, it is in fact true.

Also from the Guinness World Records, Michelle Lee Wilson gave birth to the heaviest triplets on record in July 2003. Her children weighed 8 pounds 9.4 ounces, 7 pounds 5.4 ounces, and 6 pounds 13.8 ounces at birth, and all delivered within 2 minutes of one another. These babies were carried to 36 weeks and 5 days. They, and their incredible mother, are a testament to the fact that the human body is incredibly adaptable and resilient.

## The Representation of Twins in the Media

As a child, I attended school with a pair of identical twins and naively wondered whether they could read each other's minds. Later on as middle schoolers, my friends and I devoured the Sweet Valley High books about the Wakefield twins, which later ran as a TV series (Elizabeth was the good girl, but Jessica often schemed and showed her wild side). I had limited personal exposure to twins in the real world yet viewed plenty of dramatic representations on TV (*Super Friends:* "Wonder Twin powers activate!") and in the movies (Stanley Kubrick's *The Shining* famously using the image of twins as a sign of foreboding); as a result of all the above, I perceived twins to be magical and mysterious.

Forgive the pun, but twins live dual lives in the 2 worlds of reality and in media. Each of my twins is a complex, textured individual with a unique identity, and knowing each boy with the depth of our parent-child relationship, I understand that being a twin is only one facet of their hundreds of interesting personal facets and quirks. Parenthood expands one's breadth of experience, and one of the many life lessons we learn when we become parents is that those we formerly considered under other exotic categories are now understood in a clearer light.

In the media, labels and stereotypes abound. Pop culture tends to reinforce these notions, which are not always accurate. As parents, we can recognize our own misconceptions as well as guide our children's understanding of the variety of people in this world. We can teach our kids that people are not to be generalized or compartmentalized. Each of us deserves consideration as a *person,* not as a *category.*

An important role parents play is helping our kids responsibly navigate and interpret what they see in the media, including helping your children understand how media affects their view of others in the world. Common

Sense Media (www.commonsensemedia.org) is a great family resource. Watch programming with your family and discuss, in an age-appropriate way, different characters and their representations with your kids. Are all twins jokesters à la Fred and George Weasley in the Harry Potter series, or are they good and evil counterparts such as PBS Kids Ruff and Scruff Ruffman? The good-twin–bad-twin stereotype perpetuates thinking of twins as a unit. One twin's personality is defined as how it contrasts with the other twin's personality. Most important, emphasize to your kids that each of us has a unique spirit that defines who we really are.

Not all media representations are negative or misleading, and with a little homework, parents can use TV or movies as an educational tool with their families. As an example, when Dora the Explorer became a big sister, she was surprised to gain not one but 2 new siblings (boy-girl twins). This Dora episode is a helpful way to prepare a preschooler who will soon become a big sibling to multiples. Look for positive, realistic, and age-appropriate examples of characters when watching programming with your kids. If you see a scenario that doesn't agree with your family's principles, use it as a talking point to discuss the issue. Media surround us, and parents can use media selectively and wisely to open family discussions about human behaviors and interaction.

# CHAPTER 13

# A Glimpse Into the Twin Experience

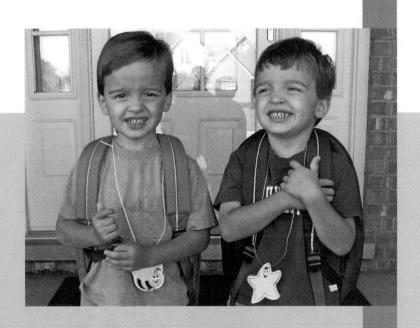

*M*y husband was asked years ago in an interview what it was like growing up as one of 8 children and he responded, "What is it like to *not* grow up with 7 siblings? It's what my experience was, so for me, it was normal." For twins or more, their personal experiences are their versions of normal. Who better to learn from than the folks who have lived life as a multiple?

## Captain Scott Kelly's Story

You've likely read about Captain Scott Kelly in the news—retired astronaut, retired US Navy captain, and former military fighter pilot. His list of accomplishments literally pushes the envelope of human progress. With 4 space flights under his belt, he is best known for being the American astronaut with the most accumulated number of days spent in space, including a record-setting, year-long mission on the International Space Station (ISS) from 2015 to 2016.

Scott's identical twin brother, Mark Kelly, is also a US astronaut. The 2 brothers are the first family members, let alone siblings or identical twins, who were accepted into the astronaut training program. Scott's autobiography, *Endurance,* shares stories from their childhood through Scott's year in space. This riveting read includes such details as the fact that the 2 brothers actually wore the same suit (loaned from one brother to the other) for their entrance interviews!

Scott and Mark are the sole subjects of the ongoing NASA Twins Study, the first of its kind to continue to examine the effects and changes to the human body in long-term spaceflight, compared with Earth. It comprises 10 separate investigators, studying 4 categories of research across multiple universities, corporations, and government laboratories. This information is critical if we are to learn what is needed for humans to travel to Mars, a much longer duration spaceflight compared with a year on the ISS. In particular, the research is looking at how knowing the genetic sequence of individuals can personalize their health care.

"When I was preparing for the press conference to announce [my 1-year ISS mission]," Scott relates in *Endurance,* "I asked what I thought was an innocent question about genetic research. I mentioned something we hadn't previously discussed: Mark would be a perfect control [participant] to study throughout the year.... Because NASA was my employer, it would [have] be illegal for them to ask me for my genetic information. But once I had suggested it, the possibilities of studying the genetic effects of spaceflight transformed the research. The Twins Study became an important aspect of the research being done on station. A lot of people have assumed that I was chosen for this mission because I have an identical twin, but that was just serendipitous."

I asked Scott about his experiences growing up and living as an identical twin. His to-the-point and often hilarious answers were both entertaining and enlightening!

**Me:** Parenting has evolved over the generations. As kids, we were not the singular focus of our parents' lives. How do you think this hands-off parenting style helped you and Mark develop as individuals, as future adults, and in your relationship with each other?

**Captain Kelly:** I think it did help. They had a free-range parenting style. I learned of this phrase recently. They said that was by design, but it was quite possibly laziness too. [*laughs*]

**Me:** Growing up in New Jersey, were you and Mark pretty much together most of the time at both home and school, or was your school large enough that you were in different classes? How did you feel about this?

**Captain Kelly:** In elementary school, we weren't allowed to be in the same class. In middle school and high school, on a rare occasion, we would be.

**Me:** You and Mark were the first relatives, let alone identical twin brothers, accepted into NASA's astronaut-candidate training program. At this level of training in both your careers, did you feel the need to actively distinguish yourself from Mark, or did this just happen naturally as time passed?

**Captain Kelly:** [We made] no conscious effort either way.

**Me:** People always compare siblings, and they especially compare twins; was this ever annoying, and if so, how did you deal with it?

**Captain Kelly:** It never bothered me much. As the only kids, we had no comparison.

**Me:** What are some of your favorite aspects of living life as a twin?

**Captain Kelly:** The spare organs.

**Me:** As a parent of identical twins myself, especially now that they are teenagers who are further defining themselves, I follow a theme of "Respect the individual while celebrating the unique twin bond." All relationships, including those of twins, evolve over the years. Were you ever competitive with each other? Are there times that competition with Mark pushed you in a positive way?

**Captain Kelly:** We were never competitive with each other, but he did push me at a critical time when it came to studying.

---

### Hard work pays off

In his autobiography *Endurance,* Captain Scott Kelly relates a story, a pivotal moment in his life, from his first year at State University of New York Maritime College. A high school friend was planning a Labor Day party, and he called his twin brother to invite him to come along. Mark Kelly responded, "I can't, I have a test coming up," followed up with, "Don't you have some sort of test coming up too? You've been in classes for a few weeks now." In fact, Scott did have his first calculus examination at the end of the following week, and Mark proceeded to yell at Scott that he should be studying the entire holiday weekend in addition to the following week, to ace the examination to help meet his lofty goals of becoming a US Navy pilot and eventually becoming an astronaut. Scott was skeptical but spent the entire weekend working every problem in every chapter, and his hard work was rewarded with the first perfect score on a test for the first time in his life. This became a turning point for Scott after which he then enjoyed the challenge of school, at this point knowing how to work hard and see that work pay off.

---

**Me:** Do you have any funny stories from yours and Mark's time at NASA, either during astronaut training or further in your careers, of cases of mistaken identity?

**Captain Kelly:** One time, an astronaut colleague called me "Mark." I said normally it wouldn't bother me, but Mark was in space at the time and he should [have] know[n] that.

One of the lighthearted twin stories Scott relates in *Endurance* involves a gorilla suit. Mark decided that Scott needed a gorilla suit on the ISS, simply because there had never been a gorilla suit in space before. Although the first gorilla suit didn't make it to the ISS because of a failed resupply mission, the second suit successfully arrived, resulting in much joy for the crew and a video Scott made with a crewmate that went viral on Earth, drawing new attention to the space station's mission and the value of the STEM fields of science, technology, engineering, and math.

# Magda and Margaret

In 1938, an expectant father from Düsseldorf, Germany, dropped off his wife who was in labor at the city hospital, for he had to travel to Münster for special university courses, a 1½ hour train ride away. Like most fathers in this era, he was not present for the birth process. On the long journey back home, he experienced "a feeling" during his travels as if something were happening. Arriving home after a long day in Münster, his parents sat him down to share the news. His wife had delivered not one but 2 baby girls named Magda and Margaret.

Magda and Margaret are fraternal twins, now 80 years old, who immigrated to the United States in 1952. Both women now live in the Chicago area, and their twin bond remains as close as ever. I had the opportunity to sit down with Magda to hear her fascinating recollections.

According to Magda, "We lived through the war, so some of the twin 'specialness' may have been lost early on, as times were rough. I was not particularly bothered that we always dressed alike when younger; that was more a function of the war and everyone being poor. At that young age, we looked very much alike, despite being fraternal. Once the war was over and school was regularly back in session, there was only one classroom per grade, so we were never split up into different classrooms. We were always the leaders of the class in such things as school processionals and parades, which were common because it was a Catholic school."

Magda and Margaret have different memories of World War II (WWII). Margaret hated going into the bunker during the air raids at the very end of WWII. Magda remembers the stories of the horrible bombings and burning of Dresden. They had different ways of dealing with those painful memories. When the women toured Europe years later as adults, Margaret refused to tour the Anne Frank home: "I don't have to go; I lived it," she said. Magda reflects, "You remember what you think is important."

After WWII ended, Magda found running errands in town for the widowed older women was a great way to earn a bit of money. There was a lack of wine bottles, and the wine industry asked families to collect bottles. Between the ages of 7 years and 10 years, Magda and Margaret had a wagon and spent 2 to 3 years collecting bottles by knocking on neighborhood doors.

When they moved to the United States at 14 years old, their family brought household goods with them, only the essentials and no books nor games, for example. Magda explains, "I was quite a collector for a while, especially German books [I found] in old bookstores when traveling," likely as a psychological consequence of being stripped of all her possessions at a younger age. Magda and Margaret dressed identically until sophomore year in high school. The day they began dressing individually was not a day of profound origins with advance planning. The big day came as a result of the girls needing to iron their own blouses each day; one day, Margaret wanted to wear a particular blouse, but Magda's was not ironed. For the first time in their lives, the girls wore different outfits to school.

Regarding these years, Magda says, "Upon our immigration to America, we were split up in high school classes and it was then that I realized how much I really liked and valued that. It was the first time in my life that I could actually achieve something on my own without direct comparison to my sister. I was able to be myself. I think it is important for twins to nourish their own identities."

Magda's now-adult daughter Diana says that, while she had a great childhood and her needs were met, there was definitely a feeling that her mom's top priority was often her twin (Diana's aunt) rather than her own children. Perhaps this is a sign that the twin bond is so incredibly strong that for these women, it ranked as highly as the mother-child bond.

Magda's husband notes that Magda and Margaret have "a sixth sense" about each other. Each can tell when the other is having issues, even across the miles. Magda, an operating room scrub registered nurse, would be working in the operating room and "have an inner feeling, not sure what it would be. When whatever it [was] was done, I would feel a release." A physical illness is one example of such "twin sense" episodes that have occurred.

Despite their twin bond, both women were fiercely independent. At the age of 12 years, the girls were separated for 6 weeks. Magda reports, "I did not miss her." Magda feels they are both unique people with completely different personalities. Magda found the insistence of others to treat the 2 girls as a unit to be frustrating. "You were never an individual unto yourself." They never had their own birthday cakes growing up, always sharing a single cake. Teachers usually had the twin girls line up first as a class, and Magda hated it. At one point, Magda improved a grade, and the feeling was "your sister has [a good grade] too, so what?" After that point, Magda decided to learn for learning's sake.

On the topic of education, Magda says, "Margaret was the smart one in Germany." Fast-forward to junior year of high school in the United States when a biography project was assigned: Magda had hers ready, but Margaret couldn't get her project going, perhaps because of bad memories growing up during WWII in Germany. This was the first time that Magda helped Margaret with schoolwork.

Magda, in the context of discussing women's limited career options at the time, stated, "I flunked shorthand 'accidentally,' on purpose, so I didn't have to become a secretary." Talking with Magda, and enjoying being in the company of her feisty, independent spirit, I wondered to myself whether her twin experience was a factor that helped her become more vocal and outspoken, to give voice to her opinions and needs.

Much has changed over 80 years. Magda's experience and wisdom gives us much-needed perspective parenting twins ourselves. Challenging times and difficult circumstances have a silver lining of building resilience and remembering what is truly important. It is emotionally healthy to keep the big picture in mind when navigating modern day twin parenting challenges.

## Lorelai and Leighton

"Are you sure you're twins?"

Nine-year-old Lorelai and Leighton are fraternal twins, although many of their classmates don't even realize they are siblings, let alone twins! They have usually been placed into the same classroom at school, and their parents and teachers have been monitoring this closely over the years for the girls' balancing personalities and independence. For their family, because their girls have independent spirits and are treated as individuals, separate classrooms aren't necessary. Their parents gratefully admit that their daughters' presence in the same classroom has made their lives a bit easier by needing to keep track of only a single classroom's assignments, projects, and routines.

Lorelai and Leighton have a single-born brother who is only 18 months younger. One of the girls shared with me that if a friend comes over to play, often "we all play with [that friend] together."

When she was in first grade, Leighton recalls befriending a classmate who happened to have a twin, a moment with which she realized that not everyone had a twin.

Lorelai's favorite part of being a twin is "It is special and rare." Leighton enjoys "having someone on my side."

The girls used to share a bedroom but then asked to be separated into 2 bedrooms when they were 8 years old. One of the sisters states that "she is messy, and I am clean."

Often twin girls, even if fraternal, can be very attached to each other. Lorelai and Leighton are perfect examples of independent spirits who are their own people yet share an incredibly special lifelong bond with each other.

# Kathy's Story

Kathy is an adult identical twin who was gracious enough to share her thoughts on living life as a twin.

**Me:** What is your favorite part of being a twin?

**Kathy:** Without sounding corny—I love everything about being a twin. As an adult, I understand how friendships come and go. I know most people probably have a best friend, but this is different. My twin, Nancy, and I have an unspoken trust and relationship. This has never wavered. We know what each other is thinking, [and] we know what each other's needs are. We have never doubted our friendship or...ever worried about it. It's simply just there. I can't even imagine not having a twin. I feel as if I have been given a special gift that not many people have.

**Me:** What is your least favorite part of being a twin?

**Kathy:** My least favorite part of being a twin is watching my older sister get very little attention compared to my twin and me. When we were little, my mother always dressed us alike, and since we are identical twins, the public was very interested in us. As adults, the 3 of us often go out together and people still approach Nancy and me to ask questions about being twins. Julie just smiles and waits patiently. She was always known as "the twins'" sister.

**Me:** Can you share a funny story about growing up as a twin?

**Kathy:** When we were born, my parents couldn't tell us apart, so my mom painted my toenail red. As toddlers, we sucked each other's thumbs. Nancy and I often switched classes in school. Nancy once went to my gym class for a whole semester so I didn't have to have wet hair in school. Not sure if I should confess, but Nancy did take a biology final for me. We went on a couple dates for each other. Nancy and I have children the same ages. Our children were 3 years old before they knew who their mom was.

**Me:** What do you wish other people knew about being a twin?

**Kathy:** We don't have weird powers, but we do know what each other is thinking and feeling. It's probably because we spend so much time together. We don't have a secret language, but we do know what each other is going to say before we say it. There isn't an evil twin. There isn't a dominant twin.

**Me:** Does it bother you when people confuse you with your twin? How do you deal with it/how do you correct them?

**Kathy:** It has never bothered me to be confused with my sister. I really don't know anything different. As an adult, if someone comes up to me and thinks I am my twin, I will usually say, "Oh, I bet you think I am Nancy; everyone confuses us." I try not to embarrass them.

**Me:** Additional thoughts?

**Kathy:** Being a twin is an honor and a joy. I feel so special that God chose me to be an identical twin. The closeness that I share with my twin brings me comfort and happiness.

## Patty and Kathy

Patty and Kathy are identical twins, now in their 50s, who were born 1 minute apart. They each weighed about 6 pounds at delivery.

Both women say, "Our parents did a great job." They give a lot of credit to their parents for treating each of them as individuals and not comparing them as they grew up.

The Jablonski twins experienced many unusual synchronicities. For example, the girls' had their first cavity in the same tooth at the same time. After college, one of the women experienced a turbulent flight on an airplane trip. Her twin, safely on the ground, had unexplained nausea at the same time. When the women compared notes later, they realized this was the first time they had experienced similar symptoms while miles apart! Both women had children at similar ages, and both had a daughter first, followed by a son. Both of their sons weighed 9 pounds 2 ounces at birth. Both had the same knee replacement surgery, a week apart from each other, on the same side.

Kathy and Patty have a lot of fun stories regarding their twin dynamic and love for tennis. "You want [your twin] to win too, but you're playing [your twin]!" They were ranked No. 1 and No. 2 players at Drake University. They both recall a challenge match that was particularly grueling, and Patty remembers feeling, "OK, you can win it," bringing the game to a close. "I never wanted to lose to anyone else, but I was OK losing to her." "We were never mad at each other." They've watched Serena and Venus Williams, professional tennis players and sisters, play each other, and state, "I could tell when the effort wasn't there," meaning that they observed the fascinating dynamic of not necessarily wanting to beat your sibling.

Patty and Kathy's partnership both on the tennis court and off it symbolizes the ideal balance of a twin relationship. Both women are unique individuals who have been respected and nurtured as such, and at the same time, they enjoy the unique, special twin bond they have with each other.

## Andrew and Ryan

I happen to live with identical twin boys, so of course I turned my microscope onto them to gain some insights into the twin experience. At the time of this interview, Andrew and Ryan were within a month of their 15th birthdays.

**Me:** What is your favorite part of being a twin?

**Andrew:** There's always someone there for you to talk to and support you.

**Ryan:** You have a helper in different situations. If you have chores, you can split up the work.

**Me:** How do you feel about the attention of being a twin?

**Andrew:** There's good attention and bad attention. It's not so fun when people who you don't know stare at you and don't say anything, or scream out loud to everyone that you are a twin. It's pretty fun when you meet other people who are twins themselves.

**Ryan:** It's not really "good attention" and "bad attention".... It's more "OK attention" and "bad attention." Many times, we will be walking down the street and random people will be staring at us, and I can hear them say, "Oh, they're twins." I'm used to it, but it's kind of annoying.

**Me:** What is your least favorite part of being a twin?

**Ryan:** You're together all the time, and it can be annoying being with the same person all the time. Sometimes you need to be with them when you don't want to be.

**Andrew:** Sometimes when you don't want to be next to someone, you have to be next to them.

We don't have enough room in our house for Andrew and Ryan to have separate bedrooms, so they share a bedroom. They would both prefer their own spaces and their own bedrooms. Oh well! They both suggested that their twin take their oldest's brother's bedroom when he moves away to college in a couple years. Neither boy wanted their brother's bedroom; they wanted to keep their current room and force their twin brother to move.

**Me:** Can you share a funny story about growing up as a twin?

**Ryan:** At a club [competitive] swim meet, one of our coaches would scribble an "R" on one of my arms with a marker and say, "OK, you're Ryan," to tell us apart.

**Me:** What do you wish other people knew about being an identical twin?

**Ryan:** People think you have a copy of yourself who is just like you. Sometimes other people tell me they wish they had their own twin who is just like them. But that's not how it works, because your twin is [a] completely different person who doesn't always agree with you.

**Me:** Does it bother you when people confuse you with your twin? How do you deal with it? How do you correct them?

**Andrew:** Yes. Usually, I will just say, "I'm Andrew." But if I'm having a bad day, I just don't say anything.

## Alex and Ian

Alex and Ian are identical twin boys who are 8 years old.

**Me:** What is your favorite part of being a twin?

**Alex:** Having someone to be with and always having someone to play with.

**Me:** What is your least favorite part of being a twin?

**Ian:** You have to share everything (like your stuffed animals).

**Me:** Does it bother you when you are called by your brother's name?

**Alex and Ian:** [*both boys, with big smiles on their faces*] No!

**Entrepreneur Twins**

Having a twin means you have a partner for life with whom to brainstorm. One of my favorite examples of adult twins inventively using their partnership and their experiences to help others is Eric and Evan Edwards, the coinventors of a type of auto-injectable epinephrine, a lifesaving medication for those with severe allergies. Eric and Evan grew up with life-threatening allergies and were clearly motivated to create a novel way to self-administer the lifesaving medication in the case of an unintentional exposure to an allergen. Eric is a physician and Evan is an engineer, and they brought their individual skills together to develop a completely new medical device.

# Multiples and the Wide World of Sports

Here are stories of physically talented twins or more who have performed at notably high levels. Hopefully, this will encourage parents of infant twins who may be in need of inspiring stories.

- The Litherland triplets, Jay, Kevin, and Mick, were born 2 months preterm and spent a fair amount of their early lives in and out of the hospital. Their mother and father both had experience in competitive swimming and thus got their boys into the pool at an early age to help develop their lungs. All 3 swam at the collegiate level at the University of Georgia. They were the first set of triplets to swim together on scholarship as Bulldogs. Jay placed second in the 2016 US Olympic time trials in the 400-meter individual medley event, earning him a spot on that year's US Olympic team.

- In the National Football League (NFL) 2017 draft, the Seattle Seahawks selected Shaquill Griffin in the third round. In the 2018 draft, the Seahawks drafted Shaquill's identical twin brother, Shaquem, in the fifth round. Shaquem made headlines for reasons other than that he was joining his twin on the same NFL team. At 4 years old, his left hand was amputated because of pain from amniotic band syndrome during his mother's pregnancy. His resilience and determination was on full display at the 2018 NFL Scouting Combine.

- Daniel and Henrik Sedin played in the National Hockey League (NHL) for the Vancouver Canucks for 17 years together, both retiring in 2018. The 1999 NHL entry draft was notable, as the Canuck's general manager made considerable strategic trades to be able to draft Daniel and Henrik as the second overall pick and the third overall pick, respectively, that year. A *New York Times* article discussing their retirement describes their play as teammates "with what sometimes seemed like a telepathic ability to find each other with passes."

- Robin and Brook Lopez are identical twin brothers who have played National Basketball Association (NBA) basketball for more than a decade. Perhaps not surprisingly, they have similar strengths and identify best with the same position—center. They played together at Stanford University but then played for different NBA teams—most likely because they fill a similar need for each team.

- The Bryan brothers, Bob and Mike, are the winningest tennis doubles team in history. Mike is 2 minutes older than Bob, and they are mirror image twins, a subtype of identical twins. Because of their mirror imagery, Bob is left-handed and Mike is right-handed, which clearly gives them a true court advantage. The Bryan brothers appeared in 76 straight Grand Slam tournaments, winning 16 total Grand Slam doubles titles.

For as much as I try to raise my identical twin boys as 2 unique, separate individuals who happen to share the same birthday, for logistical reasons (including that they also have an older brother and a younger sister), they've participated in the same sports. When they were younger, my son Ryan begged to play ice hockey in particular or any ball sport in general. With 4 kids, 2 working parents, a budget, and a community that lacked a local ice arena, we steered our twin boys toward their older brother's competitive US swimming club team.

Part of the decision to join the swim team was logistical, and part was the big picture goal of instilling lifelong muscle memory for swimming. I also loved the idea of water safety, especially because anytime we went near a body of water, whether a backyard pool, a lake, or an ocean, our kids outnumbered us. Now that my sons are teenagers, the swimming skill has afforded them employment as lifeguards, swim lesson teachers, and assistant coaches to the club swim team's younger members.

As the years have progressed, cross-country and track has become a big part of my twin sons' lives. Having swam competitively since first grade, they already had the lung capacity for distance running. As most swimmers do, they've also dabbled in club water polo (finally, a ball sport for Ryan!), but as of this writing, they haven't decided yet whether they'll join track or water polo at their high school. They're both currently high school freshmen, and in Illinois, both track and water polo are spring season sports, meaning they cannot do both. I've told them for the past couple years, "You know, one of you could do track and one of you could do water polo.... You do not have to participate in the same sport." Each time I say this, they always look at me with a combination of "That sounds like a good idea" and "Are you kidding?" incredulous at the idea of not being teammates. We'll see what they choose and support them either way.

In the meantime, we hit as many open skates and outdoor ice rinks as possible. And all winter long, we are grateful for our neighbors with whom we share a backyard, as their homemade 50 foot by 70 foot backyard ice rink gets a ton of use. Even if you choose a couple of formal sports, you can still enjoy other activities informally.

If your budget and family situation allows, by all means let your kids choose their own distinctive paths athletically and socially. If, like our family, you're navigating the realities of schedules, finances, and logistics, remember the success stories from this chapter, and be at peace with your decisions.

# CHAPTER 14

# Single Parenting, Partnership Challenges, and Divorce

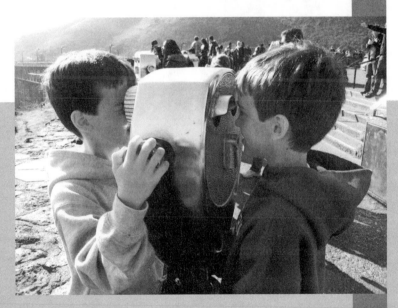

*S*tress affects relationships of all types. For any partnership, whether married or not, intense situations and stressful life circumstances affect the relationship. Examples of stressful situations include financial hardship, the loss of a job, a death in your family, moving homes, or a major illness or injury. The birth of a child, although oftentimes planned (and sometimes not), is a major life change as well, and even if welcome and hoped for, it can be stressful. The birth of twins or higher-order multiples clearly is a major life stressor, with logistical, financial, physical, and emotional challenges.

Parenting twins is parenting stepped up a couple notches. The intensity level, especially in the first couple years after your multiples' birth (add on challenges from a possibly complicated pregnancy), serves as a great stressor for partners. Poor sleep, around-the-clock tasks, and juggling personal and family needs can all take a toll. The additional mouths to feed and children to plan for creates clear financial concerns, which is ironic given that because of the intensity of parenting twins, parents likely need to modify their work hours to accommodate child care.

## Early Signs of Trouble

If you're busy and preoccupied with caring for others, working outside the home, and managing a household, it can be quite easy to ignore early warning signs that unhealthy partnership patterns are establishing themselves or are already in place. Please make sure to consult the Support, Emotional Health, and Time-savers chapter on pages 193 to 210 to streamline your responsibilities as much as possible and ensure that one parent isn't taking on a disproportionate amount of work and stress compared with the other, leading to resentment down the line.

One parent I know of, who in the process of filing for divorce, explained, "Do I think our twins caused our divorce? Absolutely not. But I would agree that the added stressors of parenting enhanced the problems, relationally and emotionally, that we already had. In a way, it was easy to ignore the relationship problems when [our] twins were younger because we were just so busy going through the day-to-day necessary responsibilities." This parent added that partners should keep the doors of communication open and be *specific* in what is requested of partners, both in sharing the household and parenting role and in what is needed on a relationship level.

Parents of twins or more may need to think creatively to carve out one-on-one time with each other. The traditional evening dinner date on a Friday or Saturday night may not be logistically feasible. When my kids were younger, I was always exhausted at this point anyway, and even if we could schedule something, I wasn't exactly in a relaxed mood ready to hang out and reconnect. For many reasons, a daytime (as opposed to evening) date may work for you and your partner. This may require some planning, enlisting the help of others, and taking a day off work, but the ability to sit for a brunch together, take a bike ride together, or do whatever your partnership would benefit from could be a game-changer.

Another parent, in the process of separating from her husband, shares, "Communication is key to any marriage, especially with multiples. Teamwork is essential to juggle all the family responsibilities. Couples lose sight of each other's personal needs and forget how to talk with each other. If a couple takes time to talk about their own needs and make[s] an effort to support each other's needs, they will have a healthier marriage, even through the tough times."

### How is love communicated?

*The 5 Love Languages: The Secret to Love That Lasts,* authored by Gary Chapman, is a good read for partners looking to strengthen their relationship. The key idea is that each of us has a preferred love language, whether it be words of affirmation, acts of service, receiving gifts, quality time, or physical touch. A pair of partners may each feel loved in different primary ways. Learning how we and our partners feel loved is a first step toward opening the doors of communication and maintaining a good relationship, long after the passion of an early romance has faded.

## Balance in Household Tasks

A lack of balance in running a household can create resentment in time. Another parent shares, "Each parent needs to be recognized for [his or her] roles in parenting. If the mother decides to stay home, she should feel as if her unpaid job is as important as her husband's paid job. It needs to be recognized that each person is contributing in some way. It is OK to praise and tell your spouse [he or she is] doing a good job too. My husband always felt this was my insecurity, and he was right. It was my insecurity, and I needed *him* to rise me above it all and make me feel like I was the supermom I desired to be."

Adds another parent, "I would say that you get caught up [in] raising kids, that in any situation, it is hard, but when you have 2 at the same time (and then another almost 5 years later) you are busy, busy, busy! You don't have the ability to set aside the time with your spouse, and when you do, you are exhausted. My ex did not understand that. He felt that I should have more to give him at the end of the day, but after homeschooling my children, cleaning [the] house, making meals, and planning outside activities, there was not a lot of time or energy left."

If you're endlessly busy, simply struggling to survive from one day to the next, it can be easy to fall into the trap of taking care of everyone else except yourself and your partner. Streamlining daily tasks as much as possible is extremely important. For time-saving and streamlining advice, see the Support, Emotional Health, and Time-savers chapter on pages 193 to 210.

# When Trouble Spots Emerge

If you and your partner notice some troubling trends appearing in the relationship, identifying these spots and communicating about them is a time-sensitive concern. Doing this early rather than after a crisis has been reached is wise. Resentment can build over time and make resolving conflicts more difficult. Speaking with an impartial third party can help identify trends and strategies for conflict resolution. Consider this option even early on, as a means to buffer your partnership from inevitable stresses and rough patches. Formal couples counseling may be helpful. You may not find a therapist with a good fit immediately, so be open to multiple attempts at finding someone with whom you both have a rapport. Looking into your house of worship's options for support for marriage or partnership is another avenue to pursue.

## Connections in Relationships

Many couples counselors use the research of Brené Brown, a professor at the University of Houston who examines vulnerability, courage, authenticity, and shame. Her TED Talks on vulnerability and shame, available online, are worthwhile for viewing when you wish to examine how you connect with others and how you view yourself.

## Taking Breaks to Refresh

Just as airlines instruct passengers to place the oxygen mask onto themselves before helping others, parents must take care of their own needs if they are to parent adequately. One of my favorite expressions is "One cannot pour from an empty cup." Don't assume your partner knows you need a break—*ask* for it. "It is very important that...spouse[s] be able to take time away from their parenting role once in a while," shares one parent. "It helps to be out talking with other friends, relieves stress, and gives a much-needed short break so they can come back feeling rejuvenated."

## Understanding the Immediate Moment and the Future

When tackling relationship struggles, it is helpful to keep the long view in mind, especially if your multiples are young. The daily logistical challenges and workload for infant twins is not the same as when your twins are in kindergarten, in fifth grade, or freshmen in high school. One parent reflects, "To make it work, you need understanding, respect, a mutual goal for the entire family, and the ability to see past the immediate moment and know that it gets different as the kids get older."

### If You Don't Feel Safe

Certain patterns are considered deal breakers, and if they are identified, you will need to take action. If you are concerned for your safety or the safety of your kids, you will need to take steps to remove yourself from your partner's presence. The National Domestic Violence Hotline is 800/799-7233, with a website at www.thehotline.org. Be advised that internet browsing can be searched, so if you are concerned for your safety, call the phone number instead.

# When Divorce Is the Decision

If the decision is made to end a marriage or partnership, how should you discuss this with your children? Keep in mind that at all ages, kids usually understand situations better than adults often give them credit for. If arguing, fights, and discord have been part of the household environment, the news won't be a big surprise. In fact, there may be a bit of relief that your family situation will be changing. Older kids who have friends whose parents are divorced may have seen it coming, although younger kids may find themselves blindsided.

Kids and teens of different ages and stages will have a varied understanding of divorce and ways of adjusting. Discussing divorce with 4-year-olds is quite different from discussions with 10- or 14-year-olds. Kids of all ages benefit from as much consistency in the daily schedule as possible. Maintain routines and keep rules and expectations as similar as possible after the transition. Shower your children with love and affection. Be present for their questions and their emotional reactions.

Children of all ages often tend to blame themselves for the divorce. Whether this is expressed to you or not, be sure to tell your kids often that this *is not their fault.* If possible, you and your partner should tell your children together. Let them know that while you and your partner will not live together anymore, this means their parents will be happier, and the transition won't change that you will always love them.

Allow plenty of time to listen to your kids. Pauses in the conversation, even uncomfortable pauses, are OK. They allow your children to think, process, and ask more questions. Especially for multiples, but even for siblings of different ages, ensure plenty of one-on-one time to make sure each child is individually heard and supported. You may find yourself surprised by how different each child's reaction is. One child may take the news quite in stride, while his twin may have a much more emotional response. They are individuals, after all.

The process of divorce, and your children's adjustment to the divorce, will evolve over time. Be present for your kids, and realize they will develop new concerns and questions as time goes on. Continue to reassure your kids that they are safe and loved. Don't underestimate the power of simply listening and being present for your children.

What does it mean to be present for your children? When a child is scared or angry, we parents are typically eager to fix an emotion or try to resolve it as quickly as possible. Consider, though, that it is helpful for kids to simply have their emotion named and *validated,* though not necessarily *fixed.* "Yes, you're angry right now. I understand. This is tough, and you feel angry about it." Then pause and allow your child to continue to express himself. This sends a message that as humans, we all feel a range of emotions, and it is *OK* to sometimes feel sad, or scared, or angry. For kids, often experiencing those emotions can be scary in and of itself. Naming and validating the feelings can be enormously helpful for a child.

**A Range of Emotions**

Depending on the ages of your children, the Pixar movie *Inside Out* can be helpful to watch as a family. The main character's family has a major move, and she experiences the range of emotions that live inside her head. It's a literal representation that we have a selection of emotions (such as happy, sad, angry, or jealous) that live inside us. The movie emphasizes that this is OK and is part of the human experience. Validating that these emotions exist and are normal will go a long way toward a child's ability to recognize and accept her own range of feelings, especially during a transition such as a divorce.

For any single parent, streamlining caregiving and household tasks is key. Consult the Support, Emotional Health, and Time-savers chapter on pages 193 to 210, and brainstorm as many creative ideas as possible. Eliciting help and troubleshooting will go a long way to help on the journey of parenting twins solo. Solo parenting is not a sprint; it's a marathon.

## Resources for Families Regarding Divorce

Books are great resources for parents and kids during a time of family transition. Some to consider are

- *Building Resilience in Children and Teens: Giving Kids Roots and Wings* by Kenneth R. Ginsburg, MD, MS Ed, FAAP, with Martha Jablow

- *A Parent's Guide to Divorce: How to Raise Happy, Resilient Kids Through Turbulent Times* by Karen Becker, MA

- *Talking to Children about Divorce: A Parent's Guide to Healthy Communication at Each Stage of Divorce* by Jean McBride, MS, LMFT

As with any life change or transition, age-appropriate books intended specifically for an audience of kids on the subject of divorce and living between 2 households can be helpful. These books help normalize the experience and serve as a great launchpad for your child's questions and an age-appropriate discussion. Some to consider are

- *Living with Mom and Living with Dad* by Melanie Walsh

- *Standing on My Own Two Feet: A Child's Affirmation of Love in the Midst of Divorce* by Tamara Schmitz

- *Why Can't We Live Together?: The Kid-Sized Answer To A King-Sized Question About Divorce* by Madison and Lucas Lovato

# Resources and Websites
# for Families With Multiples

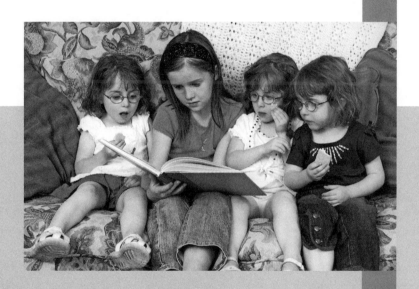

# Breastfeeding

### *New Mother's Guide to Breastfeeding*
By American Academy of Pediatrics and edited by Joan Younger Meek, MD, MS, RD, FAAP, IBCLC

### *The Nursing Mother's Companion,* 7th Edition
By Kathleen Huggins RN, MS

# General Parenting and Health Resources

### HealthyChildren.org
HealthyChildren.org is the official American Academy of Pediatrics website for parents. If your child has a mild illness or minor injury, the KidsDoc Symptom Checker tool on the website can help you decide what level of care is needed and how to provide symptom relief for minor issues you can manage on your own. A KidsDoc Symptom Checker app is available for smartphones as well.

Remember that no website or app can replace the medical care and advice of your health care professional; always address specific questions about your child's health with your pediatrician, and in an emergency situation, call 911 immediately. For those situations in which you are unsure whether you should call your doctor, the KidsDoc Symptom Checker is a useful tool to help you make an appropriate decision for your child.

### Text4baby
Text4baby is a free mobile service designed to provide pregnant women and new parents information on maintaining healthy pregnancies and babies. Parents can sign up for the service by texting "BABY" (or "BEBE" for Spanish) to 511411 to receive 3 free SMS text messages each week, timed to their due date or baby's date of birth—a helpful way to get reliable advice while on the go. Check out their website at https://text4baby.org or their Facebook page for more information.

## Meal Assistance Coordination for Bed Rest and Multiples' Homecoming

**Meal Train**
www.mealtrain.com

**CareCalendar**
www.carecalendar.org

**Take Them a Meal**
https://takethemameal.com

## Media Resources

**Common Sense Media**
www.commonsensemedia.org

Common Sense Media is a website you can use to determine whether a film is age appropriate for your kids and much more.

## Neonatal Intensive Care Unit

*Understanding the NICU: What Parents of Preemies and Other Hospitalized Newborns Need to Know*
By American Academy of Pediatrics and edited by Jeanette Zaichkin, RN, MN, NNP-BC; Gary Weiner, MD, FAAP; and Davia L. Loren, MD, FAAP

## Sleep

*Sleep: What Every Parent Needs to Know*
By American Academy of Pediatrics and edited by Rachel Moon, MD, FAAP

*Solve Your Child's Sleep Problems*
By Richard Ferber, MD

## Specific to Twins and Multiples

*Emotionally Healthy Twins: A New Philosophy for Parenting Two Unique Children*
By Joan Friedman, PhD

*Twins in Session: Case Histories in Treating Twinship Issues*
By Joan Friedman, PhD

*Healthy Sleep Habits, Happy Twins*
By Marc Weissbluth, MD, FAAP

**Multiples of America**
www.multiplesofamerica.org

*Raising Twins* **Facebook page**
www.facebook.com/RaisingTwins

**Shelly Vaziri Flais official Twitter**
@shellyflaismd

**Shelly Vaziri Flais official Instagram**
@shellyflaismd

**Shelly Vaziri Flais official blog**
www.pediatricianmomoftwins.blogspot.com

**Twins Days Festival in Twinsburg, OH**
www.twinsdays.org

*Twins* **magazine**
www.twinsmagazine.com

## Toilet Training

*Guide to Toilet Training*
By American Academy of Pediatrics and edited by Mark L. Wolraich, MD, FAAP

*Mommy! I Have to Go Potty! A Parent's Guide to Toilet Training*
By Jan Faull, MEd, and Helen F. Neville, BS, RN

## Parenting Preteens and Teens

*Untangled: Guiding Teenage Girls Through the Seven Transitions into Adulthood*
By Lisa Damour, PhD

*How to Raise an Adult: Break Free of the Overparenting Trap and Prepare Your Kid for Success*
By Julie Lythcott-Haims

## Adult Relationships

*The 5 Love Languages: The Secret to Love That Lasts*
By Gary Chapman

# Index